Ana Cristina F. Martins
Magda C. Q. Dell'Acqua
Silvia J. Papini

Profile of gastrostomy patients and the role of the carer

Ana Cristina F. Martins
Magda C. Q. Dell'Acqua
Silvia J. Papini

Profile of gastrostomy patients and the role of the carer

Gastrostomy and its implications for nursing science

ScienciaScripts

Imprint

Any brand names and product names mentioned in this book are subject to trademark, brand or patent protection and are trademarks or registered trademarks of their respective holders. The use of brand names, product names, common names, trade names, product descriptions etc. even without a particular marking in this work is in no way to be construed to mean that such names may be regarded as unrestricted in respect of trademark and brand protection legislation and could thus be used by anyone.

Cover image: www.ingimage.com

This book is a translation from the original published under ISBN 978-613-9-63616-7.

Publisher:
Sciencia Scripts
is a trademark of
Dodo Books Indian Ocean Ltd. and OmniScriptum S.R.L publishing group

120 High Road, East Finchley, London, N2 9ED, United Kingdom
Str. Armeneasca 28/1, office 1, Chisinau MD-2012, Republic of Moldova, Europe
Printed at: see last page
ISBN: 978-620-7-67481-7

Dedication

To my God for his love and eternal faithfulness.

To my husband Evandro for his love, companionship, dedication and support.

To my sons Vitor and Pedro, who brought more grace to this work. To my parents, Claudionor and Ilza, for being by my side and guiding me to victory. To my sister Ellen for her love and dedication. To my sister Elaine who never stopped believing in me.

Thank you

To Prof Dr Magda Cristina Queiroz DeH'Acqua, for her guidance, dedication, friendship, motivation and an example to be followed and admired.

To Prof Dr Silvia Justina Papini for her great attention and dedication during the formation of this work.

To my professional colleagues and friends Valdirene Cristine Corradini, Carla Letícia Moraes de Almeida, Aline Rodrigues da Silva, Lauri Dalva de Paula Diniz, Mayra Silveira Rosa Foloni, Roberta Alessandra Gaino and Jose Eduardo Castro for their collaboration and support.

To Eloísa Paschoalinotte for her availability and improvement of the statistics for this work.

To Manoela Botari for her attention and cordiality at all times.

To the family members who took part in this study for their willingness to share their lives.

To all the staff in the Nursing Department who work to make it possible for students' dreams to come true.

To the Bauru State Hospital for opening its doors and contributing to this research.

To all the people who directly or indirectly contributed to this master's thesis.

SUMMARY

Summary

Patients with malnutrition and cerebral palsy seen at the AIPEG outpatient clinic (Interdisciplinary Outpatient Clinic for Children with Encephalopathy and Gastrostomy) at HEB (Bauru State Hospital) require a gastrostomy to help with feeding due to dysphagia and are monitored by a multi-professional and interdisciplinary team. This quantitative, cross-sectional, descriptive and exploratory study looked at the profile of carers and patients at this outpatient clinic and described the difficulties encountered by these family members/caregivers at home. After being approved by the research ethics committee and signing an informed consent form, the family members/carers of the patients at AIPEG (Interdisciplinary Outpatient Clinic for Children with Encephalopathy and Gastrostomy) were approached with a questionnaire and answered open and closed questions. An analysis of the patients' medical records was also used as a data source. Data was collected between January and June 2012. The sample consisted of 50 patients and their respective family members/carers, 60.00% of whom were female, 70.00% white and with an average age of 11.43 years. The medical diagnosis of all the patients (100.00%) was cerebral palsy and 91.17% had malnutrition. The majority of patients (92.00%) had undergone surgical gastrostomy. With regard to the carers, 98.00% were female, with an average age of 40.82 years, 70.00% were white, 86.00% of the relatives/carers were the patients' own mothers and the average income was 2.32 minimum wages. As for the difficulties most frequently reported by family members/caregivers, there was a report of the ostomy tube coming out, with a prevalence of 84.00%, and 68.00% of family members/caregivers reported the occurrence of skin lesions. Gastrostomy is a procedure that helps with the patient's clinical condition, helping family members with home care, who prefer siliconised tubes at skin level (button). It is clear that although the service offers an adequate structure, with a competent multidisciplinary team and even receiving training, family members need new strategies in health education guidelines, so that they can proceed more safely, with fewer clinical complications and emotional support.

Keywords: Nursing, Gastrostomy, Home care, Gastrointestinal intubation.

PRESENTATION

Ever since I was a child, I saw in myself the desire to help other people, perhaps because I was the first child and had to help my mum with the housework and looking after my two sisters.

I think that from this time onwards, caring was introjected into my desires, which led to my choice of profession.

I went to university at the Sacred Heart University in Bauru, doing everything that was necessary: classes, internships, work placements, presentations and in 1998 I graduated, to the great pride of my parents.

The care given to the individual increasingly caught my attention, as did my admiration for the teachers who helped us in the best way possible to grasp knowledge.

The desire for nursing research had also been present since I was an undergraduate and in order to be included in this context, I was thinking of studying for a master's degree. I remained in the world of work, in the hospital field, for a while, but I saw the opportunity to realise my desire.

My first job in 1999 was at the Hospital de Base in Bauru, where I spent four years in charge of clinical patients with neurological diseases or patients requiring neurosurgery.

After this period, I went to work at the Bauru State Hospital (HEB), through a public competition. I worked in various sectors until, in 2009, I was assigned to the outpatient clinic as a nurse, and also to be part of a support group for children with encephalopathy. This service is called AIPEG (Interdisciplinary Outpatient Clinic for Children with Encephalopathy and Gastrostomy) and I noticed a very special question that needed a scientific answer.

Today, I believe that after approximately 14 years in the profession as a nurse, I am able to carry out this study. In this process, I think that God has only now allowed me to take up my master's degree, because he has plans for me. Certainly, life is a process, and after maturing on some issues, I am able to perceive important problems in the world of work and thus make efforts to systematically resolve them. I feel happy and challenged to seek knowledge in my work context, where I work with children and their families who present an important demand for care, the object of my work process in the outpatient clinic.

CHAPTER 1

INTRODUCTION

Working in an outpatient clinic with patients who need the care of a specialised interdisciplinary team leads us to reflect on the complexity of the health/disease relationship imposed on service users and their families. In clinical situations where a gastrostomy is used, the majority of patients with Cerebral Palsy are patients who need to be cared for and at this time require actions with specific competences from the multi-professional team, in order to attend to the patient and the families who are actively part of this complex daily routine. Faced with this reality, this chapter of the study was constructed to provide theoretical concepts to guide the actions and challenges that will be experienced by patients, their families and members of the healthcare team.

1.1 Gastrostomy

Access to the lumen of the stomach and upper small intestine is often obtained by inserting nasal or oral probes. These procedures are usually indicated for decompression of the digestive tract and/or food support for periods not exceeding one month. If there is a prolonged need for digestive decompression or food support, gastrostomy is recommended: a more advantageous alternative to nasogastric probing because it is more comfortable, allows greater patient mobility, does not interfere with breathing and the physiological mechanisms for cleaning the airways.[1]

In circumstances where gastrostomy is impossible or contraindicated, jejunostomy is an alternative that can be used for prolonged nutrition in patients who are unable to consume orally, such as elderly patients or those with compromised nutritional status. It is the preferred alternative in comatose patients, as the gastroesophageal sphincter remains intact, and regurgitation can occur with nasogastric meals, which is less likely with a gastrostomy.[2]

Gastrostomy is a surgical procedure that establishes access to the lumen of the stomach through the abdominal wall. The access routes usually used are by conventional "open-heart" surgery called laparotomy or by an endoscopic procedure called Percutaneous Endoscopic Gastrostomy (PEG). [3]

Despite the great advances represented by parenteral nutrition, the enteral route is still the first choice for nutritional support in patients with a functioning digestive tract, but who are unable or unwilling to eat orally. Randomised clinical studies compare the efficacy of parenteral nutrition and enteral nutrition, taking into account complications, infections, time of use, cost, mortality, among others. The efficacy and safety of the enteral route has been shown to be greater when compared to the parenteral route. Among other complications, there is a significant reduction in the risk of serious infections. [4,5,6]

The possibility of feeding a patient through a gastrostomy can be used in a variety of situations, both in hospital therapy and at home. Various acute and chronic illnesses can benefit from gastrostomy feeding, which is indicated in up to 90% of cases of reduced oral intake, usually neurodegenerative processes, repetitive bronchoaspiration from food or obstruction due to tumours in the oropharynx, neck or oesophagus, dysphagia. [7]

The first successful gastrostomy was performed by Verneuil in 1876 and until 1980 the placement of the gastrostomy tube was carried out by conventional surgery under general anaesthesia. From 1980 onwards, the endoscopic technique was described and presented by Gauderer and Ponsky, which simplified it and in some specialised services it is performed in the outpatient clinic [8,9].

1.1.1 Surgical gastrostomy

There are various types of gastrostomy used for surgical procedures, such as the Stamm and Witzel type (temporary and permanent), the Janeway type (permanent) and the percutaneous endoscopic gastrostomy (temporary). [10,11]

A. Surgical techniques

- Stamm type: among operative gastrostomies, the Stamm is the most widely used, successful, simple, quick and easy to perform. [11] The Stamm gastrostomy is the most widely used technique for inserting a gastric tube, as it requires a small laparoscopic incision. [12]

The procedure is carried out with the patient in the supine position, through a small supraumbilical median incision. The gastrostomy site corresponds to the anterior wall of the stomach, close to the great curvature, between the body and the gastric antrum. The catheter is introduced through a small opening previously made in the body of the stomach, and a purse-string suture (2-0 or 3-0 non-absorbable thread) is used. After confirming the proper position of the catheter by aspirating the gastric contents, the suture is tied and two or three more sutures are made so that the posterior suture invaginates the anterior suture, thus forming the serous path. From there, a counter-opening is made, about 3 to 5 cm from the laparotomy, to externalise the catheter. Once the catheter has been externalised, the appropriate fixation (gastropexy) of the anterior gastric wall to the parietal peritoneum adjacent to the counter-opening hole is carried out. This fixation is done using four simple points (north, south, east, west), in an attempt to prevent gastric secretion from leaking into the peritoneal cavity. Finally, the catheter is fixed to the skin and the laparotomy is closed in planes. [13]

-Witzel type: this is a modification of the Stamm technique, consisting of the construction of a longer serous tract. The patient's position and the access route to the abdominal cavity are the same as for the previous technique. The catheter is introduced into the gastric lumen and secured with a single purse-string suture. From there, the catheter is placed on the gastric wall following the longitudinal axis of the stomach and the anterior wall is pleated over the catheter using a 4 to 8 cm long seromuscular suture. The catheter is exteriorised by counter-opening, the anterior gastric wall is fixed to the parietal peritoneum as in the Stamm technique, and the anterior gastric wall is closed to the parietal peritoneum as in the Stamm technique, finally closing the laparotomy by planes. Although devised to reduce the extravasation that occurred in the Stamm technique, the Witzel technique did not provide any satisfactory advantage; on the contrary, there was even a greater propensity for extravasation around the catheter, as well as a longer operative time and greater gastric deformation. [3]

* **Stamm and Janeway type:** Stamm and Janeway gastrostomies require an upper abdominal median incision or a transverse incision in the left upper quadrant. The Stamm procedure involves using a concentric purse-string suture to attach a probe to the anterior gastric wall. A counter-opening is created in the left upper quadrant of the abdomen as an access for the gastrostomy. The Janeway procedure requires the creation of a tunnel, called a gastric tube, which is exteriorised through the abdomen to form a permanent stoma. [10]

1.1.2 Percutaneous Endoscopic Gastrostomy (PEG)

It can be reported that the GEP (Percutaneous Endoscopic Gastrostomy) technique, compared to surgical gastrostomy, has several advantages, including: (1) speed of execution, (2) shorter hospital stay, (3) lower cost, (4) avoids laparotomy, (5) does not require general anaesthesia and the use of a room in the operating theatre for most patients. [3]

A. Endoscopic technique

Patient preparation includes fasting for 8 hours, prophylactic antibiotic therapy the day before the procedure and checking basic laboratory tests (blood count, electrolytes and coagulation). The procedure is usually carried out in the endoscopy room, under sedation associated with local anaesthesia, which is well tolerated and lasts around 15 to 20 minutes. [3]

a. Pull (puncture) technique: This is currently the most widely used. Performed by two doctors simultaneously, an endoscopist and a surgeon, it consists of:

* A conventional endoscopy, with the patient in a horizontal dorsal decubitus position, to rule out any pathology that might contraindicate the procedure. The endoscopist hyperinflates the gastric chamber, forcing it closer to the abdominal wall. [3]

* Digital compression of the gastric wall by the surgeon, following the guidelines for the preferred location, which are in the left hypochondrium, 3 cm

to the left of the midline. The site is visualised by the endoscopist, who guides the surgeon to the most suitable place to perform the puncture. [9]

*   Antisepsis and anaesthesia are carried out on the site to be punctured in the abdominal wall, and then the catheter is punctured until it can be seen penetrating the gastric chamber. [3]

*   A nylon thread is passed through the catheter, which is grasped by the endoscopist with polypectomy forceps and pulled into the patient's mouth. [3]

' The gastrostomy tube is tied to the nylon thread and this is pulled by the surgeon until the tube is externalised through the abdominal wall, which is done retrogradely, i.e. passing through the oral cavity, oesophagus and finally the stomach. A small incision is made in the skin for the probe to pass through. [3]

*   The tube has a dilatation at its end called the internal ring (in its intragastric portion) which does not allow it to exit the stomach, and an external fixation ring which together keeps the gastric wall and the abdominal wall coupled. As there are no stitches to perform the gastropexy in this technique, final maturation occurs between the seventh and tenth postoperative day. [3]

b. Push technique: The main difference is that the probe does not pass through the oral cavity and is not contaminated by the flora of the oropharynx. It is inserted directly into the gastric chamber after positioning a guide wire through a trochanter similar to the one used in laparoscopic surgery. It can be performed under radiological control. [3]

c. Push technique with fixation: Firstly, two sutures and fixation are performed transfixing the gastric wall with traction of the gastric chamber through the sutures and subsequent passage of the truncater and positioning of the probe. There is currently a commercialised kit that greatly simplifies the method first described by Hashiba. [14]

- The tube is fixed in the gastric chamber using a balloon filled with water. The advantage of this method is that it prevents the tube from dislodging in agitated, confused or paediatric patients, as well as avoiding contamination of the tube by the bacterial flora of the oropharynx or passage through tumours located in the path between the mouth and the abdominal wall. [15] In cases where ascites is present, the use of sutures greatly reduces leakage, allowing the procedure to be carried out if absolutely necessary, for example for gastric drainage in patients with peritoneal metastases. [3]

In recent years, the percutaneous endoscopic gastrostomy technique has become the procedure of choice for many patients because, as well as being less expensive, it generally has fewer complications, although some studies indicate that open gastrostomy and GEP (Percutaneous Endoscopic Gastrostomy) have an equivalent preoperative risk. [12]

1.1.3 Indications for gastrostomy

A.   Gastric decompression

Gastric decompression can be achieved by means of a temporary gastrostomy, which is occasionally recommended as a complement to major abdominal operations for which gastric stasis, prolonged "adynamic ileus" and digestive fistulas are anticipated. The procedure is indicated for patients with chronic obstructive pulmonary disease, psychotic patients, agitated patients and elderly patients who wish to avoid the discomfort and risks of using a nasogastric tube. [1]

B.   Temporary Food

Indicated when access to the digestive tract is temporarily impaired for recovery and maintenance of nutritional status: gastric stenosis, oesophageal cancer and mega-oesophagus, and possibly in prolonged coma. [1]

C.   Definitive Gastrostomy

As a palliative therapy for patients with unresectable malignant neoplasms of the pharynx and oesophagus, for whom there are no favourable conditions for endoscopic or surgical transtumoral intubation, and neurological diseases such as cerebral palsy, dementia, amyotrophic lateral sclerosis, sequelae of strokes, Parkinson's disease, dysphagia and others affecting tongue, pharynx and oesophageal motility: cerebral palsy, dementia, amyotrophic lateral sclerosis, stroke sequelae, Parkinson's disease, dysphagia and others that affect the motility of the tongue, pharynx and oesophagus and compromise swallowing and nutritional status. [1]

1.1.4 Contraindications to gastrostomy

Before GEP (Percutaneous Endoscopic Gastrostomy) insertion, selected patients must be carefully assessed as to whether the procedure is indicated. Elderly patients requiring GEP (Percutaneous Endoscopic Gastrostomy) are more prone to medical comorbidities, which are vital in determining the suitability and timing of GEP (Percutaneous Endoscopic Gastrostomy) insertion; patients with severe respiratory diseases are very fragile to the sedation required for endoscopy. The inability to bring the anterior gastric wall into juxtaposition with the abdominal wall, which can be the result of previous gastric resection, ascites, hepatomegaly or obesity, are important contraindications, as well as bleeding, peritonitis, oesophageal and pharyngeal obstruction and severe acute illness. Contraindications to GEP (Percutaneous Endoscopic Gastrostomy) include neoplasms, inflammatory diseases, gastric and abdominal wall infiltration and immune system deficiencies. [16,1]

An important factor in limiting any percutaneous gastrostomy insertion is a history of previous surgery on the upper abdomen, with the potential for adhesions and structures, such as the colon interposed with the stomach and abdominal wall. Perforation of the colon, which can go unnoticed for many days, is a well-described complication of all percutaneous techniques. Under these circumstances, a Stamm gastrostomy should be performed through an incision in the left upper quadrant. [1]

Table 1 describes the indications and contraindications.

Table 1: Indications and contraindications for GEP*.

Indications	Relative indications	Absolute Indications
Nutritional support (> 30 days).	Inability of the gastric wall to approach the abdominal wall	Impossibility of moral dilation or ablation to insert the device.

	(visceromegaly, ascites, obesity, previous surgeries).	
Neurological disease, Gastric decompression.	Impediment of abdominal wall puncture in the epigastric region (wall injury, coagulopathy).	Obstruction.
Motor dysphagia (collagenosis, stroke**).	Impossibility of passing the	Previous total or subtotal gastrectomy.
	endoscope (stenosis, trismus).	
Mechanical dysphagia (peptic, caustic, tumour and actinic stenosis).	Portal hypertension, distended loops, ventriculo-peritoneal shunt, ascites, peritoneal dialysis.	There isn't.
During the treatment of head and neck tumours	Inability to handle and care for.	There isn't.
Re-administration of bile secretion (fistulas).	There isn't.	There isn't.

*PGEG, percutaneous endoscopic gastrostomy. **CVA, Cerebral Vascular Accident. Source: Pelosof AG. Percutaneous endoscopic gastrostomy. In: Kowalski, Luiz Paulo et al. Manual de condutas diagnósticas e terapêuticas em oncologia. 2 ed. São Paulo: Âmbito Editores, 2002. p. 156-159. [17]

Another drawback of gastrostomy tubes of all types is that they generally don't hang down, making it difficult to aspirate and assess residual gastric volumes.[12]

1.1.5 Complications

Gastrostomy can be performed by laparotomy, videolaparoscopy or percutaneous endoscopy (PEG), and is located in the left hypochondrium. Its purpose is gastric decompression and feeding and it has complications such as leakage of gastric contents around the tube, skin irritation, foreign body granuloma formation, pyloric obstruction by the tube balloon and others. [18]

The main complications were defined as those requiring laparotomy, blood transfusion or radiological intervention due to catheter migration. The minor complications were: obstruction of the tube, inadvertent removal of the tube, leakage around the ostomy, local or systemic infection requiring antibiotics. [19]

Table 2 describes the most frequent complications and their definitions:

Table 2: Definition of complications

Complications	Definitions
Displacement of GEP*	Any inadvertent removal of the GEP device*
Peritonitis	Examination consistent with progressive intra-abdominal inflammation
Organ damage	Organ or tissue damage
Unplanned procedure	Unexpected need procedures that require facilities with hospitalisation.
Complications	**Definitions**
Haemorrhage	Bleeding related to the GEP site* requiring intervention.
Surgical site leak.	Need for intervention due to extra-abdominal leakage.
Probe migration	Change in mental healthGEP* from their place of origin.
Surgical site infection	Celluliteorabscessrequiring antibiotic therapy.

*GEP, percutaneous endoscopic gastrostomy. Source: Brewster BD, Weil BR, Ladd AP. Prospective Determination of percutaneous endoscopic gastrostomy complication rates in children: Still a safe procedure. Surgery. 2012 oct, 152(4): 714-721. [20]

For a better and more didactic visualisation, we present the table below 3 with the complications of GEP*.

Table 3: Complications of GEP*

Minor complications	Major complications
Leakage	Early loss of the probe
Peri-sternal infection	Peritonitis
Obstruction	Aspiration
Distant migration	Drilling
Persistent pain	Gastro-colic fistula

*GEP, percutaneous endoscopic gastrostomy. Source: Wiggenraad RGJ, Flierman L, Goossens A, Brand R, Verschuur HP, Croll GA, Moser LEC, Vriesendorp R. Prophylactic gastrostomy placement and early tube feeding may limit loss of weight during chemoradiotherapy for advanced head and neck cancer, a preliminary study.Clin Otolaryngol 2007;32(5):384-90. [21]

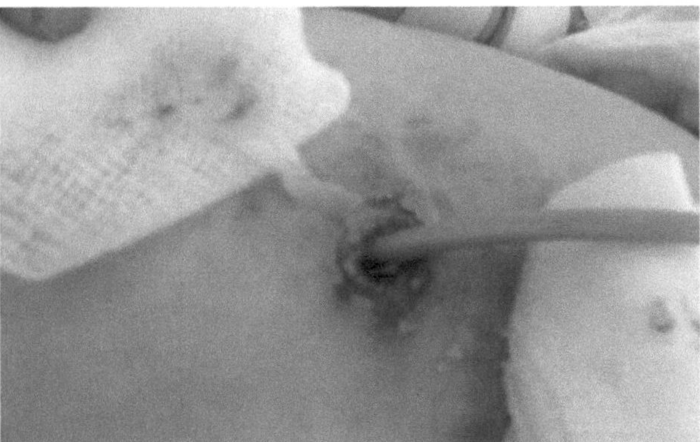

Figura 1: Patient using foley tube and mother reporting extravasation of gastric contents through perigastrostomy

Source: Personal collection: photo taken at the AIPEG (Interdisciplinary Outpatient Clinic for Children with Encephalopathy and Gastrostomy) Nursing Consultation at HEB (Bauru State Hospital).

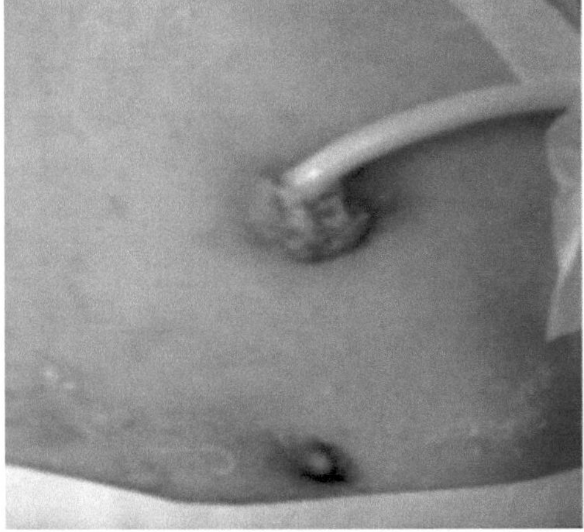

Figura 2: **Patient using a Foley tube and with a granuloma**

Source: Personal collection: photo taken at the AIPEG (Interdisciplinary Outpatient Clinic for Children with Encephalopathy and Gastrostomy) Nursing Consultation at HEB (Bauru State Hospital).

Care for the most frequent complications can be seen in table 4.

Box 4: **Complications of GEP*: causes and actions for resolution**

Problems	Causes	Actions
Necrotising fasciitis.	Necrosis of the superficial surfaces.	Broad-spectrum antibiotic therapy and surgical debridement.
Haemorrhage in the	Injury to a proximal	Compression producing

gastric mucosa puncture area.	vessel.	haemostasis, increase traction of the tube and if it doesn't stop, remove the tube and perform coagulation endoscopic.
Bronchoaspiration.	Aspiration of stomach contents due to reflux from the stomach.	Avoiding postural treatment. Apply the correct feeding technique. When it happens , suspended feeding, respiratory physiotherapy and the administration of prescribed antibiotics.
Irritation or infection around the starling.	Excessive pressure on the starling.	Adjust the distance between the base of the probe and the stoma.
	Lack of hygiene around the starling.	Clean the spout according to the guidelines. Underneath the base of the probe, place a gauze pad in contact with the skin and change the dressing daily.
	Outflow of gastric liquid.	Changing dressings daily.
Obstruction of the probe.	Administer undiluted medication into the tube.	Water should always be administered after diets and medicines. Pass 50 ml of water through the tube with a syringe. If this is not enough, have the probe replaced
Probe output.	The probe goes outside either accidentally or voluntarily.	Tell a doctor before 24 hours have passed. Place foley probe temporarily.
The probe doesn't turn all the way round.	Probe attachment.	Turn and push the probe in gently. If it doesn't turn, tell a doctor.
Nausea and/or	High osmorality.	Proper dilution of the formula.

vomiting.	Excessively rapid infusion.	Return to the correct infusion rate.
	Lactose intolerance.	Administer lactose-free diets.
	Excess fat in the diet.	Use low-fat diets.
	Hyperosmolar solution.	Use an isotonic diet and/or diluents hypertonic.
Diarrhoea.	Lactose deficit.	Supply lactose.
	Poor fat absorption. Cold diet.	Use low-fat diets.
Constipation.	Scarce administration of liquids.	Administer fluids in adequate quantities.
	Insufficient fibre intake.	Increase your fibre intake.
Periostomy granulomas.	Granulation tissue proliferation in starling.	Tissue resection and cauterisation.

*GEP, Percutaneous Edoscopic Gastrostomy. Source: Ruiz ABF, Castillo SG, Lucendo AJ. Percutaneous endoscopic gastrostomy: an update on indications, technique and nursing care.Enferm Clin. 2011; 21(3):173-178. [7]

1.1.6 Pre- and post-gastrostomy care and follow-up

Nursing care in terms of patient techniques and procedures has been used for a long time, involving the actions and knowledge of the carer towards the person being cared for. All patients must be informed of the processes and new habits they will have to adapt to, as well as the materials that will be made available to them. [23]

In preoperative nursing care, it is necessary to ascertain the type of procedure that will be carried out, laparotomic or endoscopic, in order to initiate specific guidance and care. [3]

A. The main aspects of pre-operative nursing care [3]

• Determine the patient's and/or family member's ability to understand and cope with the surgical experience they are about to undergo;

• Explain to patients and their families that the aim of the procedure will be to meet nutritional needs;

• Clarify doubts about the temporary or definitive procedure;

- Assess the condition of the patient's skin and whether they have comorbidity factors that may delay the healing process;
- The nurse responsible for preoperative supervision must not forget to keep the patient fasting for 8 to 12 hours in order to reduce the risk of aspiration and consequent complications;

R Perform oral hygiene with a 0.12% chlorhexidine solution before the procedure (when using a percutaneous gastrostomy endoscope) and perform a trichotomy if necessary.

B.   The main nursing care in the post-operative period [3]

- Explain to the patient and/or family member during their hospitalisation all the procedures that will be carried out;
- Keep the headboard elevated by 30° in order to facilitate digestion and minimise the risk of bronchoaspiration;
- Observe the characteristics of the perigastrostomy skin;
- Apply 5x5cm gauze around the gastrostomy tube in the immediate post-operative period in order to promote absorption of gastric juice peri-probe, preventing possible skin lesions;
- Administer filtered water through the gastrostomy tube as prescribed by the doctor, starting with a volume of 30 to 60 ml gradually, six hours after the procedure;
- Make sure there are no liquid leaks around the gastrostomy tube;
- Observe and record fluid tolerance according to the prescribed infusion;
- Perform abdominal auscultation, confirming the presence of hydroaerial noises before starting the diet on the 1st postoperative day. If the patient shows no discomfort after the initial administration of liquids, release the diet;
- Make a note and immediately notify the doctor in charge if there is abdominal distension or vomiting;
- Administer the diet at room temperature, making sure to check the expiry date, the patient's name and the volume to be infused;
- Handle the probe with a clean technique to prevent unwanted infections;

A Aspirate before starting the diet and check for the presence of gastric residue, considering it significant if the volume aspirated is greater than 250 ml or consult the institutional protocol. If this occurs, it is recommended to pause the diet for a period of 4 hours and then repeat the procedure;

• Adapt the medication prescribed by gastrostomy tube, avoiding crushing the medication and replacing it with syrups or solutions, in order to improve the bioavailability of the drug;

• Observe the viscosity of the medicine, if necessary dilute with filtered water;

• Rinse the gastrostomy tube with 30 ml of filtered water before and after administering each diet or medication;

• Clean the area around the gastric stoma daily with soap and water while showering, to prevent dirt from accumulating on the skin;

• Make 360° rotational movements with the gastrostomy tube every day in order to avoid the tube sticking to the gastric wall, granuloma formation and peri-stoma tissue necrosis;

• Observe daily for the presence of secretion or gastric juice per gastrostomy tube that could damage the skin;

• Avoid jerking on the probe to prevent displacement and/or accidental removal;

• Check the size of the probe, taking care not to pull it too far to avoid necrosis of the gastric stoma;

• Check and write down the demarcation number of the gastrostomy tube, always keeping the number that was chosen when the tube was inserted;

• Perform oral hygiene three times a day, using a soft-bristled toothbrush, to minimise colonisation of the oropharynx;

• Check the correct routes of administration of the diet, water and drugs, avoiding rupture of the balloon if the tube contains it;

• Treat the skin or stoma according to the established institutional protocol or at the doctor's discretion.

C.   Drug treatment for the skin.

There are treatments with medication and care (prescribed by the doctor responsible for the patient) that are used when skin irritation or granuloma occurs, such as: [18]

•   If the skin is irritated by any kind of leak, prevent it by adjusting the button or balloon and apply antacids to the skin. Place the contents of a suspended antacid in a container for 1 hour. Remove the liquid from the top and apply the thickened antacid paste from the bottom of the container to the skin. If the irritation worsens, you can use a barrier protector, which should be changed as often as necessary, usually lasting three or four days.

•   If a granuloma appears around the gastrostomy opening, it should be treated. The formation of granulation tissue is a common occurrence. It is the result of the presence of a foreign body (probe), which stimulates the production of inflammatory epithelial tissue. Treatment consists of cauterising it with a topical application of a silver nitrate stick.

1.1.7 Types of probe

The patient has contact with three types of probe and at three different times after surgery. At the time of surgery, the Pezzer probe is used, which is kept in place for up to three months and then replaced by the Foley probe, and after two months this is replaced by the Button\Mic-key® skin-level probe.

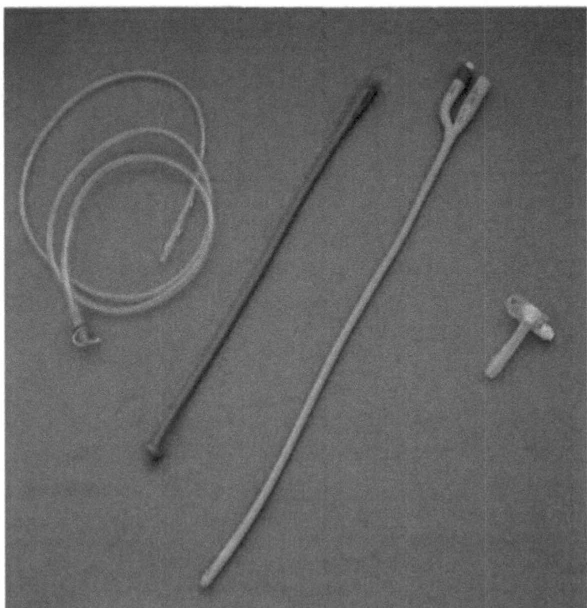

Figura 3: Probes used in HEB* (in sequence: gastric probe, Pezzer, Foley and **Button\Mic-key®**).

Source: Personal collection: photo taken at HEB*
* HEB, Bauru State Hospital

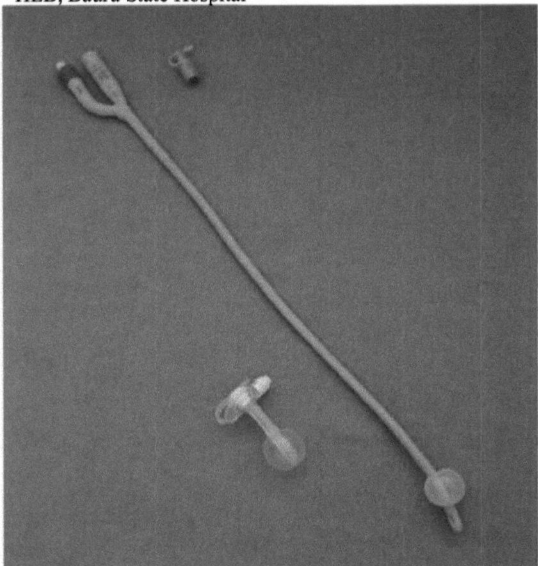

Figura 4: Foley and Button\Mic-key® probes used in HEB*.
Source: Personal collection: photo taken at HEB* of the probes used (at the initial part of the Foley, the end

These inflatable balloon tubes, used to replace the

original gastrostomy tube (Pezzer), are available in various models.

Ordinary Foley probes can be adapted for use as replacement probes. To do this, an external retainer must be fitted to prevent internal migration of the probe. The retainer can be made from a 3 cm to 4 cm piece of latex or silicone tubing, with two aligned and symmetrical transverse holes through which the probe will pass. [24]

In addition, an adapter should be placed at the inlet end to allow the connection of feeding equipment and its closure when not in use. Although Foley probes are regularly used as replacement probes, their material of construction (latex) has been associated with allergic reactions, as well as frequently showing granulation tissue formation and dysfunction due to repeated balloon ruptures caused by early degradation of the material, corroded by gastric acid. [24]

Buttons are gastrostomy devices that are fitted at skin level and were developed by Gauderer and collaborators[25] with the intention of avoiding the long length of gastrostomy tubes in children and outpatients, as well as reducing frequent replacement tube changes. [24]

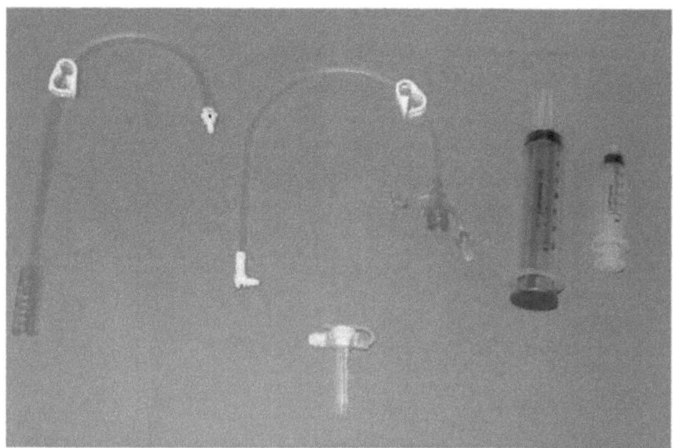

Figure 5: Button\Mic-key® probe used in HEB*.

*HEB, Bauru State Hospital. Source: Personal collection: Kimberly-Clark button probe kit
(Mic-Key) used at the HEB outpatient clinic*. Materials: extensions, skin-level probe and syringes.

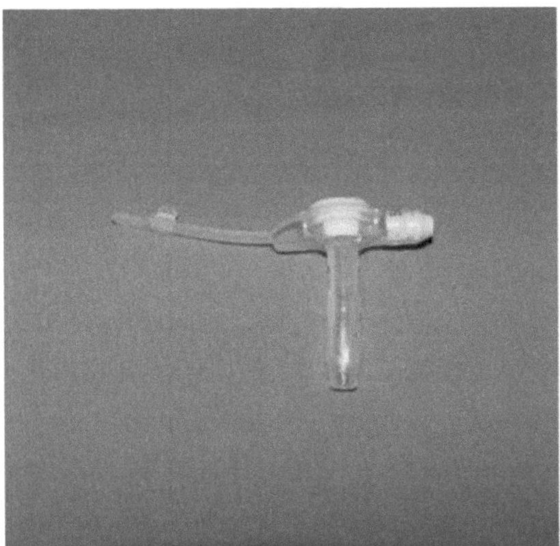

Figura 6: Button\Mic-key® probe used at HEB*

*HEB, Bauru State Hospital. Source: Personal collection: Kimberly-Clark button probe (at skin level) (Mic-Key)

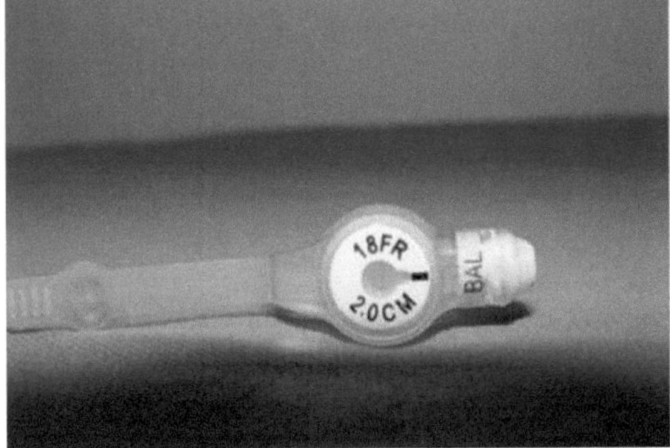

Figura 7: Button\Mic-key® **probe** used at HEB*

*HEB, Bauru State Hospital. Source: Personal collection: Button probe measuring 18FR X 2.0cm

Made of silicone or polyurethane, there are models with ballooned or fixed (but deformable) internal retainers. As they are not adjustable, they are available in a variety of lengths.

wall thickness in the gastrostomy tract before the device is ordered. [24]

Generally, the family member prefers this tube because it improves the family routine, making it easier to care for the device and the patient.

25

1.2 Cerebral palsy

The initial definition of the term cerebral palsy (CP) emerged during Freud's neurological phase, when he studied Little's syndrome or illness, which in 1843 and later in 1853, described a disease characterised by muscular rigidity, predominantly in the lower limbs, and caused by different disorders caused by asphyxiation of the newborn (NB) during birth. [26]

More specifically it can be said that CP (cerebral palsy) is a non-progressive syndrome of brain damage caused by factors operating on an immature nervous system, manifesting itself at birth or in early post-natal life, essentially showing an irregular disturbance of voluntary movements and often revealing associated deficits or disadvantages - intellectual, convulsive, sensory and educational.[26]

CP (cerebral palsy) is also known as a form of Chronic Non-Evolving Encephalopathy (CNE) in which motor disorders predominate[27] and the most frequent cause of decreased muscle strength in infants is "atonic cerebral palsy".[28]

It is no easy task to determine the incidence of CP (cerebral palsy), precisely because of the difficulties in establishing uniform diagnostic criteria and because it is not a notifiable disease. [26]

Even in First World countries, statistics vary. In England and the Scandinavian countries, in the 1950s, the incidence of CP (cerebral palsy) was estimated at 1.5 cases per 1,000 live births, while in the United States it ranged from 1.5 to 5.9/1,000. Today, in the United States, there are estimated to be between 550,000 and 600,000 patients with CP (cerebral palsy). [26]

In Brazil, the estimated incidence of CP (cerebral palsy) is likely to be higher because the conditions of pre- and perinatal care are satisfactory for only a small proportion of the population and the majority are poorly cared for.[26]

Here, infant mortality is higher and, therefore, the survival of premature and low birth weight newborns (NB) would be lower, leading to a decrease in the occurrence of CP (cerebral palsy). It's a logical reasoning, but this conclusion will have to be proven with further research [26].

However, growth and nutrition disorders are common secondary health problems in children with cerebral palsy. Cerebral palsy is the most common physical disability in children and affects 3.6 / 1,000 children. [29]

To make it easier to understand this pathology, below is a description of the 3 types of CP (cerebral palsy) that exist.

A. Spastic Cerebral Palsy

This section will discuss the forms of spastic cerebral palsy which account for % of all cases of CP (cerebral palsy) and have the following clinical types: tetraplegic, hemiplegic and cerebral diplegia. **a. Tetraplegic form**

This is the most common type, according to the Danish authors. [30] It is a very severe form, surpassed in this respect only by the so-called rigidity forms which, strictly speaking, represent more severe forms of tetraplegia.[26] Clinical manifestations are generally observed from birth, although the severity of the condition increases as the child grows. [26]

What happens is that there is an improper distribution of muscle tone, with relative hypotonia of the limb muscles and hypotonia of the head and trunk erectors. As families are impressed by the fact that the child can't hold its head up at the normal time, around three months, patients are referred to as flaccid, when in reality they already show clear signs of spasticity, especially when handled.[26] **b. Hemiplegic form**

According to the experiences of the Danish authors, this form occurs in around 20% of cases of CP (cerebral palsy)[30] and should be noticed from the first days of life, but in practice this is not always the case. In many cases, particularly those where the motor impairment is not very severe, families only take the child for a consultation after a few months of life, when they notice that the child is using the limbs of one hemibody. [26]

The motor deficit is much more evident in the second half of the year, when the activity of the upper limbs becomes richer and more varied and the patient begins to use the lower limbs to stand, crawl and walk.[26]

There is hypertonia in flexion of the upper limb and in extension of the lower limb, the foot rests on the toes, which become deformed and in vicious positions due to the retraction of the calcaneal tendon and these changes in the anatomy of the foot will, over time, make the gait even more defective, especially when the child walks fast or runs. [26]

c. Diplegic form

It occurs in 17.7%[30] and it is not easy to diagnose this type accurately at first. In many patients, motor and tone disorders predominate in the lower limbs, while the upper limbs are little affected.

However, the neurological examination will show clear signs of difficulty in executing more precise movements. [26]

The neurological picture is characterised by motor impairment of the lower limbs. In the first half of the year, there is often a delay in passing the stages of head and trunk control and there is almost always a delay in sitting or staying seated. [26] **B. Athetosis**

It was found with a frequency similar to that reported for diplegia, representing 16.9 per cent of the cases studied by the Danish authors. [30] The incidence of this form must vary greatly from one country to another, depending on the care provided to the newborns, as in most cases the aetiology of this form is linked to severe neonatal jaundice, which in around half of these cases is associated with asphyxia. [26] In this case, bilirubin encephalopathy manifests itself from the first month with intense hypertonia in extension, which causes the NB (newborn) to assume the opisthotonus position, with an accentuation of the tonic - cervical reflex, which lasts for several months, instead of attenuating and disappearing during the second month, as is observed in normal children. Patients never assume a sitting position and remain in bed with severe hypertonia in extension, which is accentuated during manipulation and emotional fluctuations. Swallowing and chewing are difficult, in many cases never developing, verbal articulation is dysarthric and difficult to understand. [26]

C. Ataxic form

It is rarer, accounting for less than two per cent of the total seen in the literature[30] and the picture is dominated by static and kinetic incoordination. Patients have asymmetrical action tremors, ataxic gait and dysarthric speech. Muscle tone is variable but dominated by hypotonia, with no signs of spasticity. [26] **D. Mixed forms**

Some of the aforementioned manifestations are combined. The most common of these is athetosis with tetraplegia and ataxia, although the semiology is complicated by the overlapping of manifestations that are confused.[26]

E. Rigidity

A not uncommon form, notable for its extreme severity, which should be better understood as a severe form of tetraplegia.[26] **F. Flaccid form**

It is uncommon and one of the most severe, with intense motor impairment and very limited development of intelligence, reflexes are not very clear and the cutaneous-plantar reflex is usually in flexion. Most of these cases don't develop speech and end their days in hospitals or organisations for the severe forms. [26]

Children with CP (cerebral palsy) often grow poorly. As a result, these children are growing further and further behind normal children. The reasons for poor growth are multifactorial and include nutritional, hormonal, physical and neurological causes. However, it seems that most poor growth is related to acute and chronic malnutrition at various points throughout life. [31]

Malnutrition is strictly related to inefficient, inadequate and insufficient feeding; while remediable to a certain extent, this unsatisfactory feeding often cannot be overcome. Consequently, in children with CP (cerebral palsy), usually severe, malnutrition is often treated by using a gastrostomy, ignoring inadequate oral feeding. [31]

A significant contributor to poor growth in children with CP (cerebral palsy) is poor nutritional status. Malnutrition occurs when a child is unable to ingest and/or absorb the necessary nutrients due to feeding difficulties or shortages, or when the child's needs, due to illness or increased metabolic rate, exceed what they can or are able to consume. Malnutrition in children with CP (cerebral palsy) is often caused by poor oral motor function, which impairs the child's ability to consume the calories and nutrients needed to support growth. [32]

Dysphagia caused by neurological diseases that mainly involve the first two phases of swallowing, which is then defined as oropharyngeal dysphagia, is a frequently encountered problem with a strong social impact. [33]

In order to detect dysphagia, a videofluroscopy examination is carried out, which is a radiological investigation based on the recording of fluoroscopic images that appear on the monitor of an X-ray machine while the patient is swallowing a radio-opaque bolus; in this way, the aspiration or penetration of food out of the oesophagus and stomach can be visualised.[33]

Many children who are referred for feeding and swallowing assessments undergo both a clinical assessment and a swallowing study (videofluroscopy), particularly when aspiration and penetration are suspected. These conditions are of concern because they jeopardise the child's health. [34]

Newborns with congenital anomalies and/or severe neurological impairment often cannot swallow after birth. In these newborns, oral feeding is associated with hypoxaemia and aspiration pneumonia, which is a serious complication reported in up to 20.00% of this population of patients with CP (cerebral palsy). Considering this, the establishment of an enteral feeding route is mandatory, either through the insertion of a nasogastric tube or by performing a surgical or endoscopic gastrostomy. [35]

It is because of the importance of the care required for children with gastrostomies, and the intrinsic need for the family member and the health team to work together, that we will address the specific topic of care, care within the confines of the home, concepts about the multi-professional team and nutrition.

1.3 Caring

Caring has always been present in human life as an essential element of existence. The dimension of technological care, in various measures, has also been and still is part of civilisations, applied in everyday life and in healing practices.

The term care is derived from the Latin "cogitatus", the English "carion" and the Gothic words "Kara" or "Karon". As a noun, care is derived from Kara, which means affliction, grief or sadness. As a verb, "to care" (from carion) means "to have concern for" or "to feel an inclination or preference for", or "to respect/consider", in the sense of a bond of affection, love, care and sympathy. (36)

In the Portuguese language, the word "cuidado" is not specifically used to define the task carried out by people who looked after others in all cultures. The word brings us the idea of responsibility, it suggests attitudes and feelings that can lead to a relationship between people, in other words, a practice, a social action. This social action was commanded by symbolic representations that, until the 17th century, were linked to religion. (37)

The word care also expresses the attention that people pay to each other, regardless of their degree of kinship, and this can be a family member, friend, neighbour or even health professionals (38)

In the process of working in healthcare, professionals are exposed to various situations that impose limits, such as stress, which is a well-known feeling, especially among nurses. This is triggered by constant contact with people who are physically and mentally ill, affected in various ways. (39)

Caring for patients with incurable diseases, or with explicit seriousness, is one of the most distressing tasks for nurses. These professionals are faced with the threat and reality of suffering and death all the time. (39)

Even so, nurses in particular must be able to carry out individualised clinical assessments, and the family must be included in this context, as it is a unit that must be included in care planning. It is hoped that care models will be applied that systematise care, with a systemic and multidimensional vision, and thus be able to meet the urgent and unavoidable demands of the person in their illness process. (40)

Nursing professionals must also bear in mind the difficulties that lay people have in assimilating so much information and content that is unknown to them. [41]

This process takes into account the level of knowledge that each person has as a personal characteristic, knowing that most carers are laypeople, and that many factors will influence the establishment of care. Family members of stoma patients, the focus of this research, certainly expect to have not only the knowledge to care for their family member, but also to be supported throughout the process. [42]

It should be noted that the family has an influence on the patient's health; therefore, family-centred care should be based on the following assumptions: recognising the strength of the family as a constant in the child's life; facilitating collaboration between parents and professionals at all levels of health care; respecting and valuing the family's cultural, racial, ethnic and socioeconomic diversity; recognising the family's strengths and individualities, respecting the different coping methods; continuously share unbiased information with the family; respond to the developmental needs of the child and the family; adopt policies and practices that provide emotional and financial support; plan care that is flexible, culturally competent and responsive to the needs of the family; encourage and facilitate family and network support. [43]

With this in mind, we present some concepts about home care, which is the primary focus of attention for children with stomas.

A. Home Care

The perspective of care in the home must be considered, because in this context there are countless reports of the experiences of people with the condition and their families and/or carers who, through these actions, provide for the survival of a large number of children. Many are technology-dependent and need to manage devices and appliances. [40]

Even with the technological advances in medicine, the health system is not always able to return a healthy child or adolescent to their families of origin. In many cases, this child can bring with them a bleak prognosis, marked by the most diverse disabilities, losing sight of the abilities that characterise the notion of childhood that we all have, such as the right to run, play and grow. [44]

Thus, the degree of dependence on care and biopsychosocial support can be as variable as the diagnoses and the diversity of conditions that are currently presented in the health care context. [44]

Transition planning With advances in medicine, many children with special health needs are surviving into adulthood[45] and many providers feel unprepared to care for these patients. [46]

However, in order to care for their child or family member, the carer needs to be empowered as a carer, and for this they need to be helped. [42] Caring for someone requires everyone to understand the other person as an integral human being. The carer needs to perceive the patient's suffering and understand their moment of pain. [47]

Carers must know how to deal with their emotions, have "emotional competence", so that these do not influence their participation in care. Patience and an appropriate response to situations facilitate their participation. [41]

It is important to stress that the carer's perception of how much the care tasks affect their life and routine directly influences the activity of caring. Knowing all the difficulties that the family will encounter, the nursing team has to guide them through the division of labour at home. [41]

Families are made up of people with different personalities and life goals, so it's important to be aware of each person's individuality and uniqueness. [41]

Medically fragile children with complex care live at home and often need technological support, such as: supplementary oxygen, respiratory or cardiac monitors, mechanical ventilation, vascular access devices, and/or feeding tubes. These children are mainly cared for by their parents and often with nursing care at home. [48]

Children who are dependent on technology are affected emotionally, socially and academically and it has damaged their quality of life and their families also endure emotional difficulties, social isolation, divisions between family members and sibling rivalries. [49]

It is true that many children are dependent on others for their care, are not active participants in school and do not live independently, their care is expensive and extremely time-consuming. Many die early or require extensive care for the duration of their lives [46].

Therefore, to the extent that responsibility for care is transferred to family members, as well as the use of technologies, and this outside the domain of professionals, emotional, social and financial burdens are known to emerge, which can only be alleviated by educational actions that prioritise autonomy, acceptance and social support. [50]

Faced with this reality, we can generate new knowledge by helping to reflect on the best action for each case, with the aim of updating, renewing, simplifying and making practice and the actions involved more efficient. [51]

In view of this fact, knowing that childcare will be carried out by the family members who will take over the care, it is necessary to involve the family in this process, with intentional actions aimed at health education from the perspective of prevention and promotion. [52] Addressing concepts about multi-professional teams is extremely important when it comes to the difficulties that families face, and this is the subject of the following item.

1.4 Multi-professional team

Teamwork has been proposed as a strategy to tackle the intense process of specialisation in healthcare. This process tends to vertically deepen knowledge and intervention in individualised aspects of health needs, without simultaneously contemplating the articulation of actions and knowledge. [53]

In the literature consulted on health teams, it was noted that team definitions are relatively rare. The bibliographic survey showed a predominance of the strictly technical approach, in which the work of each professional area is understood as a set of attributions, tasks or activities. In this approach, the notion of a multi-professional team is taken as a reality, since there are professionals from different areas working together. [53]

However, teamwork does not mean abolishing the specificities of the work, as technical differences express the possibility of the division of labour contributing to the improvement of the services provided, as specialisation allows for the improvement of knowledge and technical performance in a given area of activity. [53]

Health professionals stress the need to preserve the specificities of each specialised job, but also express the need to make the division of labour more flexible, i.e. professionals carry out interventions specific to their respective areas, but also carry out common actions such as: reception, welcoming, educational groups, operative groups and others.[53]

Thus, multi-professional teamwork is a form of collective work that is shaped by the reciprocal relationship between multiple technical interventions and the interaction of agents from different professional areas through communication, the symbolic mediation of language. [53]

Teamwork takes place in the context of objective work situations in which the flexibility of the division of labour and technical autonomy with interdependence are maintained alongside hierarchical relations between the different levels of subordination, making it possible to build team-integration even in situations in which asymmetrical relations are maintained between the different professionals. [53]

Given these facts, we can say that the majority of patients who undergo procedures and need home care, whose fundamental points are the patient, the family, the family context and the carer, need a multi-professional team to offer support and care.[41]

The following are nutritional concepts that are highly relevant to understanding the reality of the patients in this study.

1.5 Nutrition

Growth and nutritional disorders are common secondary health problems in children with cerebral palsy. Physical growth is a fundamental measure of health and well-being in children, and abnormal growth can be considered a sign of a child's altered nutritional status. [29, 55]

Even under apparently good living conditions such as a suitable environment and regular medical attention, children with CP (cerebral palsy) grow more slowly than normal children. Decreased body fat and poor overall growth are common in children with CP (cerebral palsy), these changes in the development of these patients are closely related to malnutrition, which leads to an increased need for health care for these patients. [56,57]

Malnutrition jeopardises children's growth and development and can lead to irreversible damage, including to the brain. This will depend on its severity and the length of exposure, hence the importance of systematically assessing nutritional status, especially in hospitalised children.

According to the American Public Health Association, nutritional status is the health condition of an individual influenced by the consumption and utilisation of nutrients and identified by the sum of information obtained from physical, biochemical, clinical and dietary studies. It will therefore reflect the balance between balanced food intake and the consumption of energy needed to maintain the body's daily functions.

The Nutritional Status Assessment is essential for establishing intervention attitudes and aims to: identify malnourished or obese patients; quantify and classify the type of nutritional alteration; verify the effects of diseases on nutrition and metabolism, assist in risk prognosis, and monitor the effectiveness of recommended nutritional therapy.

It is therefore of fundamental importance to standardise the methodology to be used for each age group, standardising the assessment criteria used by the team. A complete assessment of nutritional status includes: medical, social and dietary history; anthropometric data; clinical and biochemical assessment.

Among the available methods, anthropometric ones, which make it possible to assess body density and stocks of lean mass and adipose tissue, as well as monitoring growth, are the most widely used for monitoring the nutritional status of children and adults.

The most commonly used indicators for assessing the nutritional status of children are weight and height measurements. Literature references are used to classify and assess nutritional status, based on percentiles by percentage adequacy[58,59] and the Z-score[60] , which relates weight for age, height for age and weight for height.

There are special situations that require specific assessments, such as correction for prematurity, Down's Syndrome, Cerebral Palsy, among others.

Krick[61] developed growth curves (P/I, E/I and P/E) after studying 360 (175 female and 185 male) children with quadriplegic cerebral palsy, with the aim of providing a growth reference standard for children with quadriplegic cerebral palsy.

Measurements were taken at the time of a visit to an orthopaedic clinic and retrospective review of medical records. Statistics were carried out to check for significant differences in relation to the National Centre for Health Statistics (NCHS) growth charts and the results of the growth charts were constructed for boys and girls aged between 0 and 10 years. [61]

Given these facts, we can say that the majority of patients who undergo gastrostomy and need home care, whose fundamental points are the patient, the family, the family context and the carer, need a multi-professional team to offer support and care. [41]

Home care for a child with a gastrostomy can make it difficult for the carer, due to its specificities and the complexity of experiencing these activities with such a dependent and significant person. It is necessary to be aware of this demand for care and to be able to reorganise the work of nurses in order to use care models that take into account the adequate preparation of these carers.

As a member of the team, you can see the importance of each team member's role, as their specific skills are complemented and the aim is to provide more comprehensive care for the child and family.

The patient in this context, with all his clinical limitations, as well as the difficulties inherent in the personal conditions of the relatives responsible for providing care, clearly justify the validity of this study.

Knowing the limits in a systematic way can help to promote care in an expanded way and offer support, guidance and health education, which can enable care with less compromise.

There was an interest in verifying and analysing how the care provided by mothers, fathers, grandparents - in other words, the main caregiver chosen in each family, according to their particular dynamics - has been carried out.

In view of the above, the purpose of this research is to seek data and information from family members, with the intention of proposing new strategies and promoting forms of communication that facilitate the approach at home.

In view of the points already made, the question for the study is: what is the profile of the patients cared for in this service, by this interdisciplinary team? And what are the demands and difficulties presented by family members or carers of patients with gastrostomy at home?

The objectives are now presented.

CHAPTER 2

OBJECTIVES

2.1 General Objective

The aim of the study was to verify the epidemiological profile of patients with gastrostomy tubes and to analyse the main difficulties inherent in the demands made by carers in their daily lives at home.

2.2 Specific objectives

• Check the profile of the patients in terms of: age, gender, ethnicity, medical diagnosis, nutritional diagnosis, weight, estimated height before, on return and in the late post-operative period of up to six months and how many types of feeding (gastrostomy or together with oral);

• To characterise carers in terms of: age, gender, ethnicity, degree of kinship, education, profession, number of people living in the same house, income, housing conditions and type of transport they use;

• To identify the difficulties faced by carers/family members in caring for gastrostomised patients at home.

CHAPTER 3

METHOD

3.1 Type of study

This is a descriptive, exploratory, cross-sectional and quantitative study to be carried out at the gastrostomy outpatient clinic of the Interdisciplinary Outpatient Clinic for Children with Encephalopathy and Gastrostomy (AIPEG) at the Bauru State Hospital (HEB), Bauru, São Paulo.

3.2 Ethical procedures

In accordance with the national and international guidelines for research with human beings of the Council for the International Organisation of Medical Sciences (CIMS) and Resolution 196/96 of the National Health Council[62] , this project was submitted to the Research Ethics Committee of the Botucatu Medical School in São Paulo.

The favourable opinion can be found in official letter no. 566/2011, with protocol CEP 4104-2011 at the approval meeting on 05/12/2011 (Annex I).

3.3 Study site

This Interdisciplinary Outpatient Clinic for Children with Encephalopathy and Gastrostomy (AIPEG) was set up in 2006 at the Bauru State Hospital (HEB), made up of professionals such as: a paediatric surgeon, a neuropediatrician, a paediatrician, a speech therapist, a psychologist, a social worker, a nutritionist and a nurse.

From the outset, the aim is to monitor children diagnosed with dysphagia with encephalopathies and with an indication for gastrostomy. This takes place with a clinical assessment carried out by all the team's professionals, and once the videofluoroscopy examination for dysphagia has been confirmed, the patient goes on to be surgically programmed for gastrostomy, and everything is reported in the electronic medical record.

In order for the team to work properly, it follows the description of HEB's rules and routines, and each member has their own duties: - Nutritionist "provides care for all patients who have or will have a gastrostomy, helping to indicate the gastrostomy procedure. The patient will be accompanied by the nutritionist during hospitalisation until discharge and then followed up by the team."[63]

•   The speech therapist "assesses the patient's swallowing and suggests an alternative long-term feeding route. After the gastrostomy, the patient will be followed up in the group, assessing the possibility of introducing and maintaining the partial oral route."[63]

•   Social Worker "attends through interconsultation, whenever the team deems it necessary or at the request of the patient's carer"[63]

•   Psychologist "is responsible for the psychological care of all family members and/or carers of patients before and after gastrostomy. Psychological instruments (interview scripts) and techniques will be used, as well as psychological interventions according to the needs of each case."[63]

•   Paediatric surgeon "assesses patients with a potentially reversible disease, or an incurable disease with long survival potential, or seriously debilitated terminal patients. He selects patients for the procedure (gastrostomy), with all the tests ready and the family's consent, and excludes patients with contraindications; contraindications are discussed on a case-by-case basis, with assessments by the whole team" (63).

•   The paediatric surgeon is also responsible for "providing post-operative guidance in relation to gastrostomy. Observe for signs of gastroenterological complications related to the gastrostomy".[63]

•   A paediatrician is responsible for "providing paediatric medical care to all the patients in the group, with dietary, vaccination and preventive advice, ordering tests, hospitalisations and taking patients to the outpatient clinic with acute illnesses, as well as taking part in the discussions for the indication of gastrostomy."[63]

- Paediatric neurologist "assesses and assists in the treatment and investigation of patients with chronic encephalopathy and its complications such as spasticity, osteo-articular deformities, epilepsy, behavioural changes, sialorrhoea, sleep disorders, headaches and neuropathic pain, contributing to improving their quality of life and promoting health as a whole." [63]

- The nurse is responsible for "carrying out a nursing consultation where the patient/family/carers will receive guidance demonstrating the care of the tube/gastrostomy and changing the gastrostomy tube as prescribed by the doctor".[63]

This group of professionals meets once a week and assesses the indications for gastrostomy in children with cerebral palsy (CP) or other encephalopathies, and in this work context the idea for this research was born.

3.4 Population

The outpatient clinic has the particularity of being designated for child patients, but over the years the children have become adults and because there is no other team to do similar work for adults, the AIPEG team (Interdisciplinary Outpatient Clinic for Child Patients with Encephalopathy and Gastrostomy) decided to continue monitoring these patients.

Patients are seen by all the professionals individually and after this time the team meets and decides what will be proposed for each patient, but together, the team, family and patient often suggest gastrostomy as a therapeutic proposal.

The outpatient clinic's routine initially consisted of four appointments, with one new case each week, but currently around nine patients are seen, with one new case each week. During the study period, January to June 2012, 85 patients were seen at the outpatient clinic, of whom 50 were included in the study. Of the remaining thirty-five patients, sixteen were excluded, four patients died, two patients lost a segment, one patient was discharged and twelve patients did not attend appointments during the study period.

The study population was made up of patients with encephalopathies, gastrostomy patients with a diagnosis of dysphagia, with silent aspiration or not, and most of them under the age of eighteen; only eight were older.

The selection criterion for the subjects was that the patients should have been at least six months post-surgery and attended the AIPEG outpatient clinic (Interdisciplinary Outpatient Clinic for Children with Encephalopathy and Gastrostomy) at a scheduled appointment during the data collection period for this study.

Their carers and/or family members, who were also part of the study, were approached by appointment.

3.5 Data collection instrument

All the care provided to the patient is described and recorded in the electronic medical record, and all the professionals have access to consider what the other professionals have proposed and how they have recorded their observations, as well as the behaviours decided by the group.

The electronic medical record consists of the patient's registration number and identification. The date of the appointment is recorded, which makes it easier for all professionals to monitor decisions and all procedures carried out on patients.

Figure 8 and 9 show the screens on which this data is recorded.

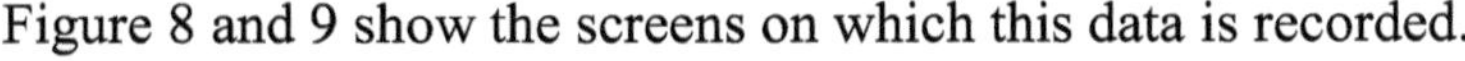

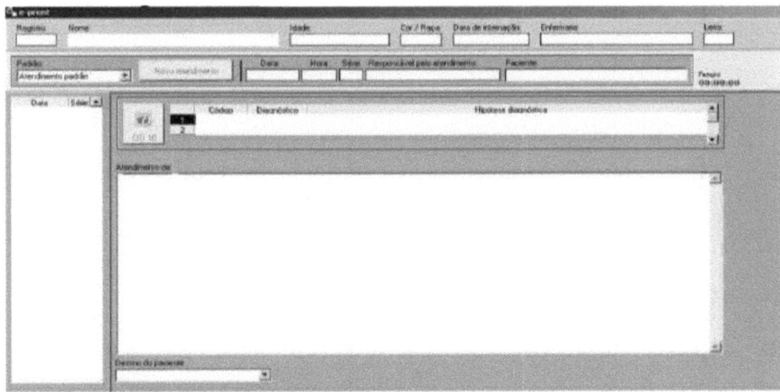

Figure 8: Electronic Patient Record

Source: Photo from the electronic medical record of Bauru State Hospital

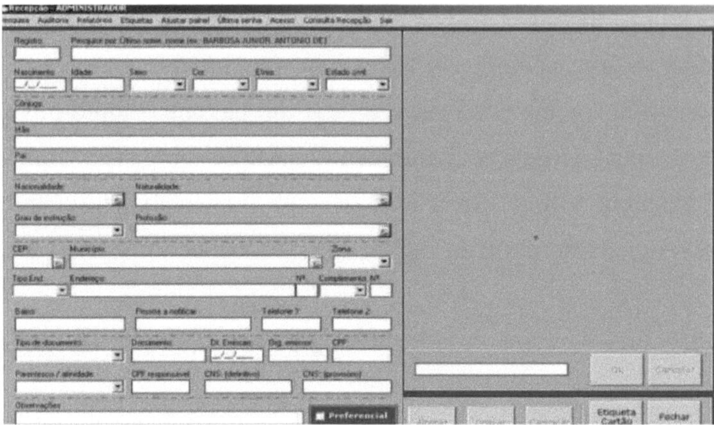
Figure 9: Patient registration

Source: Photo of the patient's personal record on the Bauru State Hospital computer system

The patient profile was collected from the electronic medical records according to the questions to be investigated in Appendix 2.

A questionnaire (Appendix 3) was administered by the researcher herself and a trained collaborator, with open and closed questions at the time of outpatient care, with the aim of surveying the demand for home care.

On the days of consultations with the AIPEG team (Interdisciplinary Outpatient Clinic for Children with   Encephalopathy and Gastrostomy), family members/carers were invited, in accordance with ethical recommendations, to take part in the study after signing the Informed Consent Form (Appendix 1). The difficulties involved in caring for gastrostomised patients at home were identified.

A free and informed consent form was given to 2 mothers who authorised photographs of their children's gastrostomies in order to visualise lesions on them.

3.6 Analysing the data

Initially, a descriptive analysis was carried out with frequency and percentage for the quantitative variables and means, standard deviation, median, minimum and maximum values.

To check the correlation between the amount of diet and the time of administration, Person's correlation was used. The analyses were carried out using SAS for Windows version 9.2, after using Excel 2007 for all the variables, and p<0.05 was taken as the level of significance.

The statistical analysis used, Person's correlation (Pearson Correlation Coefficients), for the relationship between the ml of the diets for each administration and the time of administration with p=0.0335 and R=-0.30439, showed that as the amount in ml of the diet increases, the time of administration decreases, which can cause diarrhoea in the patient.

CHAPTER 4

RESULTS

A total of 50 patients and 50 carers/family members were assessed and the results presented are related to the carers/family members' variables, professions, relationship to the patient, ethnicity, schooling, housing, place of residence and transport.

Data on patient-related variables, current tube use, occurrences of gastrostomy tube exit, occurrences of perigastrostomy skin damage, gender, ethnicity, city of residence, main medical diagnosis and nutritional diagnosis are also presented.

4.1 Data on carers

Below is the information and tables relating to the data collected from carers.

The average age in years of the carers was 40.82+/-, with a minimum of 25 years and a maximum of 70 years, and the average income in minimum wages per family was 2.32+/-, with a maximum of 4.82 minimum wages.

Table 1: Frequency distribution of the variables according to profession, relationship to the patient, education level and ethnicity of the carers. Bauru, 2012

	Variables	Frequencies	%
Professions	No activity	41	82,00
	Others	9	18,00
TOTAL		**50**	**100,00**
Kinship	Mum	43	86,00
	Grandma	5	10,00
	Others	2	4,00
TOTAL		**50**	**100,00**
Education	Complete and incomplete primary education	20	40,00
	Complete or incomplete high school.	21	42,00

	Higher education complete or incomplete.	4	8,00
	Illiterate	5	10,00
TOTAL		**50**	**100,00**
Ethnicity	White	35	70,00
	Brown	12	24,00
	Black	3	6,00
TOTAL		**50**	**100,00**

Table 1 shows the distribution of the 50 participating carers according to profession, relationship to the patient, schooling and ethnicity. It can be seen that the majority of carers (82.00%) do not work, while the other 18% are self-employed, retired, mechanics, seamstresses, drivers, day labourers, nurses and confectioners. As for the degree of kinship, there was a predominance of the mother as the main carer with 86.00% and the other 4% were the father and paternal aunt. In terms of schooling, 82.00% had secondary or primary education and 70.00% of the carers were white.

Table 2: Frequency distribution of variables according to the composition of people in the families under study. Bauru, 2012

	Variables	**Frequencies**	**%**
N°. people in families	Families of 3	15	30,00
		12	24,00
	Families of 4	11	22,00
	Families of 5		
		12	24,00
	Others		
TOTAL		**50**	**100,00**
No. of children		31	62,00
	Family with 1-2 children		
		11	22,00
	Family with 3 children	8	16,00
	Family without children		
TOTAL		**50**	**100,00**
Elderly as a member family	Families without elderly people	37	74,00
	Families with 1 or 2 elderly people	13	26,00

TOTAL		**50**	**100,00**

Table 2 shows the distribution of the variables according to the composition of the people within the families and that the number of people in the families varies from 3 to 5 people in 76%, the other 24% refers to 4 families with 7 people, 2 families with 8 people, 3 families with 6 people and 2 families with 2 people. The majority, 62 per cent, of these families have one to two children and only 26 per cent have one or two elderly people as family members. Of the 50 main carers in question, 4 are elderly and 8 families have children over 18 who are patients at the clinic. **Table 3:** Distribution of the frequencies of the variables according to living conditions, the neighbourhood where they live and the type of transport used by the families under study. Bauru, 2012

	Variables	**Frequencies**	**%**
Number of	4 to 5 rooms	31	62,00
rooms	6 rooms	8	16,00
	Others	11	22,00
TOTAL		**50**	**100,00**
	With water and electricity	50	100,00
TOTAL		**50**	**1000,00**
	With cemented floors	49	98,00
	No reply	1	2,00
TOTAL		**50**	**100,00**
	Slab	28	56,00
Cover	Ceramics	10	20,00
	Others	12	24,00
TOTAL		**50**	**100,00**
	Periphery	26	52,00
Neighbou	Centre	24	48,00
rhood			
TOTAL		**50**	**100,00**
	Public	36	72,00
Driving	Private	13	26,00
	Others	1	2,00
TOTAL		**50**	**100,00**

Table 3 shows the distribution of variables according to living conditions, the neighbourhood where they live and the type of transport they use. Of the 50 families interviewed, 62.00% live in a house with 4 to 5 rooms, the other 7 families live in 3 rooms, 1 family in 7 rooms and 2 families in 11 rooms. The absolute majority live in a house with running water and electricity.

It also shows that 56.00% of patients live in houses with a slab, while the others show that 3 families have asbestos roofing, 6 families have pvc roofing and 3 families have wooden roofing. In addition, 52.00% of families live on the outskirts and 72.00% of families use public transport.

4.2 Patient data

Below is information and tables relating to the data collected from the patients:

It can be seen that 82.00% of the patients in the study have cerebral palsy as their main diagnosis, the other 18.00% of patients have other main medical diagnoses respectively such as: Muscular dystrophy 2.00%, Dysmyelinating disease 2.00%, Dandy Walker malformation 2.00%, Microcephaly 2.00%, Extreme prematurity 2.00%, Oesophageal gastric reflux 2.00%, Cornelius de Lange syndrome 2.00%, West syndrome 2.00% and Silver Russel syndrome 2.00%.

The average age of the patients is around 11.43 years, with a minimum age of 2 years and a maximum age of 28 years.

Table 4: Frequency distribution of variables according to gender, ethnicity and city of residence. Bauru, 2012

Variables		Frequencies	%
Sex	Female	30	60,00
	Male	20	40,00
TOTAL		**50**	**100,00**
Ethnicity	White	35	70,00
	Black	4	8,00
	Brown	11	22,00
TOTAL		**50**	**100,00**
City of origin	Bauru and Jaú	23	46,00
	Barra Bonita and Lençóis Paulista	8	16,00

	Cafelândia, Dois Córregos and Lins	6	12,00
	Others	13	26,00
TOTAL		**50**	**100,00**

Table 4 shows the frequency distributions of the variables according to gender, ethnicity and the city where the patients live. It can be seen that 60.00% of the patients are female. With regard to ethnicity, 70.00% of the patients were white. The city where 36.00% of the patients live is Bauru, 10.00% of the patients are from the city of Jaú; 8.00% are from the city of Barra Bonita; 8.00% are from the city of Lençóis Paulista; 4.00% are from the city of Cafelândia, 4.00% are from the city of Dois Córregos and 4.00% are from the city of Lins, totalling 12.00% and others distributed in the DIRX region (Pederneiras 2.00%; Macatuba 2.00%; Bariri 2.00%; Arealva 2.00%; Avaré 2.00%; Agudos 2.00%; Iacanga 2.00%; Cabrália Paulista 2.00%; Promissão 2.00%; Pirajuí 2.00%; Piratininga 2.00%; Lucianópolis 2.00% and Balbinos 2.00%, totalling 26.00%).

Table 5: Frequency distribution of the variables of the type of gastrostomy performed, which ones were performed at HEB, how many days the patient was hospitalised for this procedure. Bauru, 2012

Variables		**Frequencies**	**%**
Type of procedure	Surgical gastrostomy	46	92,00
	Endoscopic gastrostomy	4	8,00
TOTAL		**50**	**100,00**
Made at HEB*	Yes	35	76,09
	No	11	23,91
TOTAL		**46**	**100,00**
Days of hospitalisation for the surgical procedure	2 to 5 days of hospitalisation	20	57,15
	Others	15	42,85
TOTAL		**35**	**100,00**

Table 5 shows the frequency distributions of variables such as: which type of gastrostomy was performed, which were performed at HEB (Bauru State

Hospital) and how many days the patient stayed in hospital for this procedure. Of the 50 patients interviewed, 92.00% underwent surgical gastrostomy, of which only 76.09% were performed at HEB (Bauru State Hospital); 57.15% were hospitalised for between 2 and 5 days for this procedure and the variable others shows that 14.28% of the patients were hospitalised for between 6 and 10 days, 8.57% of the patients were hospitalised for between 11 and 20 days, 14.28% of the patients were hospitalised for between 21 and 50 days, 2.85% were hospitalised for 72 days and 2.85% of the patients were hospitalised for 292 days due to complications with their state of health.

Of the 50 patients in the study, 72.00% did not use oral feeding concomitantly with gastrostomy tube feeding.

Table 6: Frequency distribution of the nutritional diagnosis variable for patients who had undergone gastrostomy at their first appointment with the nutritionist at this hospital. Bauru, 2012

Variables	Frequencies	%
Malnutrition	31	91,17
Eutrophy	2	5,88
Nutritional risk	1	2,95
TOTAL	**34**	**100,00**

Table 6 shows the frequencies of the nutritional diagnosis variable for patients who had undergone gastrostomy in this hospital at their 1st[a] appointment with the nutritionist. However, 1 patient was not given a nutritional diagnosis because it was not included in their medical records. However, it can be seen that 91.17% had a diagnosis of malnutrition, 5.88% had a diagnosis of eutrophy and 2.95% had a diagnosis of nutritional risk.

Table 7: Frequency distribution of the variables relating to the patient's participation in an educational institution*, receiving a diet at this institution, who administers the diet at this institution and who taught this person. Bauru, 2012

Variables		Frequencies	%
Attends an	Yes	32	64,00
educational	No	18	36,00

institution			
Total		**50**	**100,00**
You receive food at this institution	Yes	30	93,75
	No	2	6,25
Total		**32**	**100,00**
Who offers diet at this institution	Nursing	21	70,00
	Mum	6	20,00
	Others	3	10,00
Total		**30**	**100,00**
Who managed the diet	Nobody, because the employees already knew	14	46,66
	Don't know	5	16,66
	No answer	4	13,34
	Mum	3	10,00
	HEB	2	6,67
	Others	2	6,67
Total		**30**	

Examples: APAE, SORRI and conventional school.

Table 7 shows the frequencies of the variables relating to the patient's participation in an educational institution, receiving a diet in this institution, who administers the diet in this institution and who taught this person. 64.00% of the patients under study attend an educational institution, 93.75% are fed ad in the institutions, of these, 70.00% are fed by the nursing staff; with the other 10.00% being the teachers who administer the diet and one mother not being able to say whether it is the lactarist or the nursing staff who administers the diet. With regard to guidance on how to administer the diet in the institutions, 46.66% of the carers interviewed reported that the staff already knew how to administer diets in gastrostomy tubes, while the remaining 6.67% reported that it was the speech therapists at SORRI and the nurses at HEB (Bauru State Hospital) who taught the institution's staff how to administer the diet.

4.3 Data on the difficulties encountered by carers

Below are tables of data collected from interviews with carers and their perceptions of the difficulties:

Table 8: Frequency distribution of the variables referring to current tube use in patients, carers' reports of foley tubes, button tubes and their preference for tubes. Bauru, 2012

Variables		Frequencies	%
Current probe	Button	40	80,00
	Foley	10	20,00
Total		**50**	**100,00**
Reports on Foley	Negative points	36	72,00
	Positive points	9	18,00
	Others	5	10,00
Total		**50**	**100,00**
Button reports	Positive points	47	94,00
	Negative points	1	2,00
	Others	2	4,00
Total		**50**	**100,00**
Reports on Pezzer	Doesn't remember	23	46,00
	You've had problems	12	24,00
	Disliked	4	8,00
	Liked	5	10,00
	Little use	3	6,00
	Not used	3	6,00
Total		**50**	**100,00**
Probe preference	Button	46	92,00
	Foley	4	8,00
Total		**50**	**100,00**

Table 8 shows the frequencies of the variables relating to the use of current probes; carers' reports of Foley, button and Pezzer probes. Regarding the current use of the type of probe, 80.00% use the button type probe (probe at skin level). Regarding the use of the Foley probe, 72.00% reported negatively and the other 1 did not answer, 2 had not used the Foley probe and 2 did not remember.

With regard to the reports of the button probe, 84.00% are positive and 2.00% say that their child has never used it and 2.00% don't know what to say.

With regard to the Pezzer probe, 46.00% report that they don't remember this type of probe and with regard to preference, 92.00% of the carers interviewed prefer the button-type probe.

Table 9: Distribution of the frequencies of the variables relating to carers regarding training in tube care and handling of the diets received. Bauru, 2012

Variables		Frequencies	%
Training			
	Yes	44	88,00
probe care	No	6	12,00
Total		**50**	**100,00**
Diet handling	Yes	46	92,00
training	No	4	8,00
Total		**50**	**100,00**
Comment on	Yes	40	80,00
whether the	No	10	20,00
guidance was			
sufficient			
Total		**50**	**100,00**

Table 9 shows that the majority of carers received guidance on tube care and diet handling and considered the training they received to be sufficient.

Table 10: Frequency distribution of variables in relation to complications regarding the use of the tube. Bauru, 2012

Variables		Frequencies	%
Ostomy tube	Yes	42	84,00
exit	No	8	16,00
Total		**50**	**100,00**
What you did	He went to an	19	45,23
after you got	emergency service		
out of your	Put it back	14	33,33
ostomy	I capped it with gas and	5	11,91
	went to S.S.		
	Others	4	9,53
Total		**42**	**100,00**
Occurrences	Yes	14	28,00
of diarrhoea	No	36	72,00
after probing			
Total		**50**	**100,00**
Diet	Yes	6	12,00
aspiration	No	44	88,00
Total		**50**	**100,0**
Emesis due to	Yes	22	44,00
the tube	No	28	56,00
Total		**50**	**100,00**
Occurrences	Yes	18	36,73

of reflux	No	31	63,27
Total		**49**	**100,00**
Occurrences of probe obstruction	Yes	12	24,00
	No	38	76,00
Total		**50**	**100,00**
Occurrences of skin damage	Yes	34	68,00
	No	16	32,00
Total		**50**	**100,00**
What you did with the injury	Cleaned well and used ointments	16	47,05
	Sunbathing	5	14,70
	Oily lotion, based on AGE vitamins	4	11,77
	Saline solution	2	5,89
	Others	7	20,59
Total		**34**	**100,00**

Table 10 shows that 84.00% of patients had their ostomy tube removed. Of these, 45.23% sought a health service immediately, the others reported that: 2.38% a friend helped; 2.38% requested the emergency service by telephone and were attended to; 4.76% went to the health service with the tube in hand and with an occlusive dressing on the gastrostomy.

Of these 50 patients, according to their carers, 72.00% did not have diarrhoea, 88.00% did not have aspiration, 56.00% did not have emesis, 63.27% did not report reflux, in this case one carer did not answer, 76.00% did not have tube obstruction, 68.00% did not have periostomy skin lesions after cleaning, another 2.94% reported having cleaned the lesion well,00% had periostomy skin lesions after placement of the tube and of these patients 47.05% used non-specific ointments on the lesion after cleaning, another 2.94% reported having cleaned it well, another 2.94% dried it, 2.94% used or changed gases, 2.94% used boric water, 2.94% used alcohol and 5.88% used gases to keep it dry.

Table 11: Distribution of the frequencies of the variables in relation to the difficulty of administering the diets, types of diets, place of acquisition, quantity in millilitres of administration and duration of administration of the diets. Bauru, 2012

Variables		Frequencies	%
Difficulty passing diets	Yes	8	16,00
	No	42	84,00
Total		**50**	**100,00**
Moment of difficulty in passing diet	Change diet and medication to a thick consistency	4	50,00
	Others	2	25,00
	In the beginning	1	12,50
	When I wore a button	1	12,50
Total		**8**	**100,00**
Types of diets	Industrialised	45	90,00
	Others	5	10,00
Total		**50**	**100,00**
Where you buy your diet	City Hall	35	70,00
	DIR10	9	18,00
	APAE	1	2,00
	Others	5	10,00
Total		**50**	**100,00**
Millilitres with each diet administration	100ml to 200mll	34	68,00
	220ml to 300ml	16	32,00
Total		**50**	**100,00**
Time\minutes of diet administration	15 min to 30 min	13	26,00
	40 min to 55 min	14	28,00
	60 min to 90 min	21	42,00
	120 mins	1	2,00
	Others	1	2,00
Total		**50**	**100,00**

Table 11 shows that 84.00% of the carers had no difficulties administering the diet. Of the 16.00% of carers who had difficulties, 50.00% reported difficulties in changing the brand of diet and medications with a thick consistency, while the others said that they didn't know when it was difficult or that it depended on the child's position and agitation.

With regard to the types of diets, the majority were industrialised, and as for where they got their diets 54.00% were from the town halls in their cities of origin; the others in this question said that they received them from social assistance, or from the health centre, or from the government or health post, and one carer who didn't answer this question.

68.00% of carers reported administering between 100ml and 200ml at each feeding time and 42.00% controlled the administration time to between 60 min and 90 min.

As already mentioned, the statistical analysis used, Person's correlation (Pearson Correlation Coefficients), for the relationship between ml of the diets for each administration with the administration time with p=0.0335 and R=-0.30439, showed that as the amount in ml of the diet increases, the administration time decreases.

Table 12: Distribution of frequencies in relation to intercurrence variables regarding tube use. Bauru, 2012

Variables		Frequencies	%
Probe balloon	Yes	36	72,00
rupture	No	14	28,00
Total		**50**	**100,00**
Ent	Yes	29	58,00
rance	No	18	36,00
Foley for the stomach	Others	3	6,00
Total		**50**	**100,00**
Occurrence of	Yes	22	44,00
leaks	No	28	56,00
Total		**50**	**100,00**
Perigastrostomy	Yes	34	68,00
skin lesions	No	16	32,00
Total		**50**	**100,00**

Table 12 shows that 72.00% of patients have had a balloon rupture, 58.00% have had a Foley tube enter the stomach, another 4.00% report not having used Foley, 2.00% can't say, 44.00% have had gastrostomy leaks and 68.00% (36) have had skin lesions.

CHAPTER 5

DISCUSSION

This study was carried out with the aim of characterising the profile of the caregiver and the patient and analysing the difficulties reported in home care by caregivers of patients with cerebral palsy. Patients who are accompanied by a multidisciplinary team who work together to provide the family with more knowledge and comfort in caring for their loved ones.

The conceptualisation of cerebral palsy has generated many doubts, but it's important to say that as neuroimaging technology evolves, it's allowing us to discover aetiologies that were previously considered obscure. It is becoming increasingly possible to diagnose the causes more accurately, which are almost always related to chronic childhood encephalopathies due to pre- or perinatal sequelae. [64]

These patients, most of whom suffer from dysphagia, suffer from malnutrition and poor neuropsychomotor development and gastrostomy tube feeding is a frequent and essential intervention for a child who requires enteral nutrition support in order to sustain adequate growth and development. [65]

This study took into account the patients and their families followed up at the AIPEG (Interdisciplinary Outpatient Clinic for Children with Encephalopathy and Gastrostomy), held at the Bauru State Hospital outpatient clinic.

The survey approached 50 carers and their families with encephalopathies and gastrostomies.

5.1 Carers

With regard to carers, we can see that the vast majority (82.00%) do not have any professional activity, considering that these people could not work because they are responsible for caring for the patient in question and have to spend a lot of time on this. [65]

This means not being able to participate financially in the family income, because faced with the duty of caring for someone who is ill, the carer is unable to contribute to improving the family's economy. [66]

What this team advises all families going through this process is to seek the right to sickness benefit from the competent body, in these cases the National Social Security Institute (INSS), with a value corresponding to one minimum wage to supplement the family income. [67]

By submitting an application to the competent authority, supported by documents proving the patient's state of health, the patient can benefit from the resources provided by the INSS (National Social Security Institute).

However, it is not uncommon for patients to be denied benefits by the institute, even after undergoing rigorous examinations. In these cases, our team advises family members to claim their possible rights through the courts. This advice is in line with the considerations of Leite et al, who state: "we consider it advisable to propose a change in legislation so that the mother of a child dependent on technology can claim social security or welfare benefits for as long as the situation of technological dependence persists. This measure would certainly alleviate a situation of great family stress".[40]

Regarding the degree of kinship, 86.00% of the cases found that the carers were the patients' own mothers, and as reported by Machado[68] "it is known that affection between the carer and the family member is essential, but it does not guarantee competence in caring, the need for support and guidance for family members who provide loving care and thus make it possible for their relatives to recover and be treated at home is clear", even though they don't have the necessary knowledge of the disease and its burdens, they set out, out of a feeling of unconditional love, to look after their own. This demonstrates the predominance of mothers and women as carers, as only one man (a father) reported being the main carer. So, as in the other articles we researched, mothers are the focus of this study. [68, 40,66]

We should also appreciate what Cabral says: "The family is then faced with a new child, which leads to the need for family members, especially the mother, to incorporate knowledge and practices that are alien to their daily lives and lifestyles. The home welcomes the child with its artefacts, medicines and equipment, which are added to the toys and games of the child's life," reinforcing that the statistics are in line with the literature. [60,65]

As for schooling, 42.00% of these carers have completed or incomplete secondary school. This implies a significant reduction in their labour capacity, as they have difficulties in developing a profession due to their poor education, with the exception of 9 carers (18.00%), who are self-employed concomitantly with caring for their relatives.

The table below shows the profile of the carer carried out by a qualitative study by Susin et al, and showed a similar level of education to this study. [70]

It also reveals that the majority of carers are mothers and that most of them do not work, which shows a similarity in this study.

Table 13: Socio-environmental data

Family Income	One minimum wage 4 (30.77%)	Two minimum wages 5(38.46)	Above three minimum wages
Mother's age	Average 29.30 years Variation between 21 and 40 years		
Mother's marital status	Lives with the child's father 10(76.92%)	No partner 3 (23.08%)	
Mother's schooling	Incomplete primary education 4 (30.77%)	Complete primary education 2(15.38%)	High school 7 (53.85%)
Mum's working day	Full-time 2(515.38%)	Doesn't work 10 (76.92%)	Other 1(7.69%)
Father's schooling	Incomplete primary education 4(30.77)	Completed primary school 4(30.77)	Completed high school 5 (38.46%)
Father's working hours	Full-time 9(69.23%)	Doesn't work 3 (23.07%)	Other 1(7.69%)

Source: Susin FP, Bortolini V, Sukiennik R, Mancopes R, Barbosa BLDR. Profile of patients with cerebral palsy using gastrostomy and effect on carers. Rev. CEFAC. 2012 Sep-Oct; 14(5):933-942[70]

It's worth emphasising that a better level of education helps them to understand their family member's illness, to know how to take care of them, to be trained and to learn the instructions given during consultations.

As a result, we would point out that illiterate carers find it more difficult to understand the guidelines, and should be approached in a different way so that their understanding matches the seriousness of the case, because they even administer controlled medication according to the doctor's prescription, as Costa et al say "anticonvulsants are drugs widely used by patients with CP (cerebral palsy) to control seizures, and carbamazepine and valproic acid are described as the most common".[71]

However, the emotional burden borne by the carer when they see their child undergo this procedure contributes to a deficit of understanding, regardless of their level of education, because caring for the patient at home also causes concern, as we can see: "the phenomenon of family dependence in relation to carrying out activities of life is not a problem.
daily life generates a great deal of worry and causes changes in the rhythm of life for carers". [68]

With regard to family income, we can report that the average family salary is around 2.32 minimum wages. 51.02% earn less than 2 minimum wages, 34.70% earn more than 2 minimum wages up to 3.50 minimum wages and 14.28% earn more than 3.50 minimum wages and we can relate this to Susin FP, et al who say: "the data collected shows a low monthly family income since the majority, 69.23%, earn up to two minimum wages, as well as a family configuration where the father works and the mother does not work in the labour market. [70]

When observing the living conditions of these patients, we see that in order to carry out care, especially related to gastrostomy and feeding, sufficient supplies must be available, including physical, financial and social resources to provide care. [10]

In Perissé's dissertation we see that: "for Nightingale the comfortable environment promotes health and she understood the manipulation of the physical environment as the main component of nursing care. She identified ventilation and heating, light, noise, bed and bed linen, cleanliness of rooms and walls, and nutrition as the most important areas that nurses could control. He also believed that as well as fresh air, the client needed direct sunlight. He realised that it has very real and tangible effects on the human body". [23]

With regard to housing conditions, we found that the majority live in good conditions, in properties with 4 to 5 rooms, with running water, electricity, cemented floors and with a prevalence of slabs as roofs, making it possible to better sanitise the environment and also helping to organise the daily routine for carers and their families, as can be seen from Machado's report, which states: "care routines support the dynamics of families and fill the days of carers. These activities are necessary to keep the home environment in order and provide the family member with the conditions to be sanitised and to eat in the correct quantity and at the correct time". [68,23]

Having good hygiene conditions prevents the proliferation of live pathogenic microorganisms ready to take up residence in a person who is favourable to the proliferation of these microorganisms, given that patients like ours are the perfect culture medium for the proliferation of microorganisms, as they don't move, often have postural deformities and, above all, fragile health. [10]

With regard to the location of the homes, we observed that they are predominantly situated on the outskirts of the city, in 52.00% of cases; this leads us to infer that families may have some difficulties getting their patients to the city centre, where establishments supplying inputs, materials, food, clothing and other products necessary for family life are usually located, since they often need special transportation due to the use of wheelchairs and/or because they are bedridden patients.

However, we would like to point out that in the majority of the reports on travelling, 72.00% of the cases involved public transport.

Precisely to meet this need, especially when the patient is not taken care of in this respect, the whole group, especially social assistance, guides and helps the family member to assert their right as a citizen and their humanitarian value before society and before the authorities responsible for the patient's wellbeing, demanding more safety in their transport.

In terms of ethnicity, 72.00% of the interviewees are white, with an average age of 40.82, with a minimum of 25 years old and a maximum of 70 years old. It is worth noting that there are 4 elderly women who are the main carers of these patients.

With regard to the family, 54.00% are made up of up to 4 people, and 62.00% of families have between 1 and 2 children, which shows that after having a sick child.

In 26.00% of the families, there are between 1 and 2 elderly people, which often puts an overload on the carer, who as well as looking after the sick family member, has to assist the elderly person who also requires specific care.

We can see in the IBGE (Brazilian Institute of Geography and Statistics) study that: "The perception of a poor state of health leads to greater use of health services among the elderly. In 2003, elderly women declared a worse state of health than men, except among the elderly aged 80 and over, where the trend is reversed, with men declaring a worse state of health than women." As we can see in the graph below.[72]

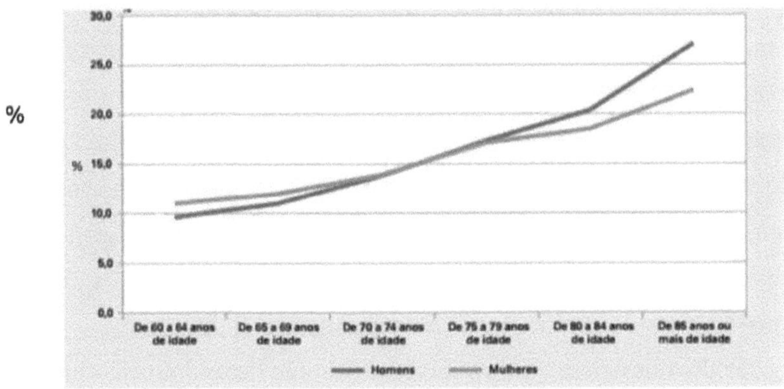

Figure 10: Proportion of elderly people reporting poor and very poor health, by age group, according to sex - Brazil - 2003

Source: IBGE (Brazilian Institute of Geography and Statistics), National Household Sample Survey 2003[72]

In our clinic, grandparents take on the role of parents when the latter are absent due to personal problems such as drugs, divorce or death, becoming the main carers.

Of the 50 carers interviewed, 4 are elderly, 1 is their mother and 3 are grandparents. This shows that the elderly still have a great deal of responsibility in the family, especially given the increase in life expectancy, which is in line with IBGE data that states: "Life expectancy from the age of 60 increased between 1999 and 2003 in all age groups, for both men and women; however, the life expectancy of women exceeds that of men and this fact explains, in part, the higher proportion of elderly women in relation to men."[73]

5.2 Patients

In terms of ethnicity, 70.00% were white, 8.00% were black and 22.00% were brown; as for gender, 60.00% were female and 40.00% male.

We can see that in Margre's study of sociodemographic data, the participants were 22.70% patients and 77.30% carers, with an average age of 28.7 years (10.60%) and of the patients who took part in this study (5 patients), 60.00% were female and 40.00% male, with no ethnicity identified. Although this is a small number to compare, it should not be overlooked as it is an important study in analysing the profile of cerebral palsy patients reaching adulthood. [74]

This patient's place of residence varies according to the cities in the DIR X (health service vacancy regulatory centre) region, such as Bauru, which accounts for 36.00%, Jaú, Barra Bonita, Lençóis Paulista, Cafelândia, Dois Córregos, Lins, Pederneiras, Macatuba, Bariri, Arealva, Avaré, Agudos, Iacanga, Cabrália Paulista, Promissão, Pirajuí, Piratininga, Lucianópolis and Balbinos.

Over time, as the outpatient clinic's services become better known, children from other regions come in search of help, to the point where family members from other Brazilian states migrate to our hospital centre. Of the patients under study, 1 (one) came from the north-east of the country to improve his treatment, according to his family.

This shows that families, no matter how difficult they find it, go to a health centre in order to treat their sick relatives. Thus, we can report that the existence of this service is of paramount importance to the population, and is necessary to support these families.

Health programmes and strategies have been inspired and put into practice, both for health services and for health professionals, who are eager to care for this type of patient, as we can see in the literature. According to Milbrath et al, "the SUS should represent the construction of a new institutional framework. In which the citizen has the right to health and with the principles of universality, equity and integrality of health actions".[75]

However, we cannot fail to note that, according to Mlibrath's qualitative study, "the testimonies show that the families were not contemplated by the hierarchisation and comprehensiveness of the health services.[74]

Milbrath also states that "It is not enough to give the family guidance and indicate more complex care for the child with cerebral palsy. It is essential that health services and actions make it possible to put this guidance into practice, providing feedback to assess the results obtained. Furthermore, as far as possible, the services should establish interaction to discuss the progress made, as well as jointly planning new care strategies that cater for this group."[74]

Therefore, this reality, which this study shows is happening all over the country, reflects the search by families in other places for special centres that provide adequate treatment for these children who need technology to survive.

A hospital or health centre with an organised, interdisciplinary and multi-professional team can make a difference to the lives of these families, and this is what our team is doing with the support of our institution.

Of our patients, 82.00% have cerebral palsy as their main diagnosis and the other 18.00% have cerebral palsy as a secondary medical diagnosis, so we can conclude that 100.00% of patients have cerebral palsy. This predominance is due to the type of pathology we treat, which is most often followed by problems with swallowing, requiring a gastrostomy.

As Fung[76] says: "A significant contributor to poor growth in children with cerebral palsy is poor nutritional status. Typically, malnutrition occurs when a child is unable to absorb necessary nutrients (due to feeding difficulties or shortages) or when the child's needs (due to illness or increased metabolic rate) exceed what he or she can consume. Malnutrition in children with cerebral palsy is often caused by poorly functioning oral muscles, which impair the child's ability to consume the calories and nutrients needed to support growth."[76]

This disease, as has already been pointed out, brings with it a number of aggravating factors: problems with eating, getting around, communicating, due to the weakness of their health, interacting with their family and with society. [26]

An illness that can lead to various other situations in which families, faced with difficulties, tend to disintegrate if there is no support, especially emotional support, as Glat and Duque report "the birth of a disabled child disorganises the family in such a way that it is necessary to make roles more flexible in order to prevent family ties from breaking down for good and thus make it possible to accept the new family member". [77]

In a way, although we can't say that it's a physically mutilating disease, in its manifestation with neurological deficits that result in the absence or reduction of movements, communication and thoughts, this disease hurts the feelings of parents who follow their children's lives, which interferes with family dynamics, parental relationships, influences the economy and emotionally and psychologically burdens the family, in many cases triggering psychiatric illnesses within the family.

Children with this type of illness should be monitored by a specialised health team to help them and their families through this process.

Often, because of dysphagia, she is unable to eat properly and needs options and means to facilitate her nutrition, and the team at this outpatient clinic suggests a surgical gastrostomy.

However, our patients are on average 11.43 years old, with a maximum of 28 years old and a minimum of 2 years old. We can, however, say at this point that the AIPEG outpatient clinic (Interdisciplinary Outpatient Clinic for Children with Encephalopathy and Gastrostomy) was set up to help children with encephalopathy, but the children in this group are coming of age.

We therefore have 8 patients in this group who have reached adulthood, and as there are no other services to meet the needs of these patients and their families, we continue their treatment so that they can survive, as we can see in Margre's study, in which he studied 5 patients with cerebral palsy with an average age of 35.2 years. [74]

As Strauss et al report, "since the 1980s, greater importance has been given to appropriate nutritional status for children and adults with disabilities, there has been early recognition and vigorous treatment of infections, as well as better technological support available in medical services".[78]

In Brazil, Guimarães mentions that "there is an increase in the life expectancy of the population in general, given the better living conditions and health care we can relate the increase in life expectancy also of these types of patients together with the technology used today".[79]

Among the patients surveyed, 92.00% underwent surgical gastrostomy, while 8.00% underwent endoscopic gastrostomy, which demonstrates the surgical profile of our clinic. However, in a review of the literature, Sleigh et al reported no convincing evidence of the benefits of gastrostomy placement in children with severe motor disabilities.[80] A subsequent clinical trial by Sullivan et al, however, has contributed to the evidence that the placement of a gastrostomy is improving nutrition and is, in fact, beneficial for the child and the family. [81]

It is notable that this surgical approach allows the paediatric surgeon to complement the anti-reflux valve surgery (cardioplasty) when necessary.

Of the 50 patients in this study, 62.00% underwent anti-reflux valve surgery (cardioplasty), of these, only 9.67% did not undergo cardioplasty in conjunction with the gastrostomy procedure and in the studies by O'Neill et al and Fonkalsrud et al it was reported that the surgical treatment of gastro-oesophageal reflux is designed to result in significant clinical improvement in neuropathic children, reducing respiratory complications and improving quality of life. [82,83]

Of the patients who underwent surgery at HEB (Bauru State Hospital), 57.15% stayed between 2 and 5 days in hospital; in a few cases there were complications. We would like to highlight a patient who was 3 years old at the time of the surgery, was hospitalised for 292 days because she had ARDS (Acute Respiratory Distress Syndrome), and is now at home dependent on oxygen therapy, requiring a mechanical ventilator on numerous occasions to help maintain her physiology.

Of the 50 patients under study, 72.00% do not use oral feeding, so 72.00% use gastrostomy feeding exclusively. This demonstrates these patients' need for gastrostomy, an excellent alternative offered to this patient profile, which is in line with the reports already presented. [75]

In the outpatient routine, the patient undergoes a clinical phonoaudiological assessment of swallowing and videofluoroscopy is performed to confirm dysphagia and penetration of food into the tracheal cavity.

We found that 91.17 per cent of these patients were malnourished, a nutritional diagnosis that is often related to low nutritional intake, but in these cases it is not the intake that harms nutrition, but dysphagia.

Because of dysphagia, carers spend the day making pasty or even liquid feeds in an attempt to provide patients with adequate nutrition, but they don't notice the silent aspiration, they don't quantify the portion expelled through the mouth and they don't correlate the various and repeated infections.

With all this, the patient's body wastes away and a state of cachexia is established, a condition that evolves with very low neuropsychomotor development, a drop in immunity and several hospitalisations to treat infections.

It is worth emphasising that in these cases, even with adequate nutritional support, patients are unable to recover their nutritional status.

These patients suffer from seizures and therefore use controlled medication.

No matter how hard the carers try to administer the medication correctly and at the right times, due to dysphagia, difficulty swallowing and the escape of oral medication, crises are often not controlled.

However, with the gastrostomy, the patient doesn't run this risk, the medication goes straight into the stomach and doesn't escape, the introduction of the tube is immediate and the reduction in crises can be seen.

Another aspect that has been verified is that 64.00% of these patients attend an educational institution (Sorri, APAE or conventional school) where they have social interaction and can learn to develop within their limits. In Brazil there is an incentive for children with disabilities to attend conventional schools, as Enumo says "The inclusion of people with educational needs in schools is a dominant proposal in Special Education and Education in general in recent decades, driving educational and rehabilitation programmes and policies in several countries, including Brazil. It demands the transformation of the school, advocating the inclusion of students with any needs in mainstream education, with schools adapting to the characteristics of the students, which leads to a break with the traditional teaching model." [84]

This is new and schools have been adapting to this new reality by providing specialised teachers and staff, such as occupational therapists and nurses.

In Margre's study, 2 patients had completed secondary school, 1 had incomplete secondary school, 1 had completed primary school and 1 attended a special school.[74] This shows both in Margre's research and in this study that even though they are debilitated, they still manage to take part in educational institutions, improving their socialisation.

In 93.75 per cent of cases, these children or patients are fed in these institutions, which is relevant data, and indicates that these institutions need to adapt to the reality of these patients by not transferring this burden to other people.

We found that of these patients, 6 mother carers (12.00%) remain outside the institution waiting for the feeding time to come and pass the diet through the tube.

These mothers don't work, but they do have other duties, such as looking after the house and other children, so these institutions must be better equipped to accommodate these patients calmly and safely.

In the institutions where the diet is given to these patients, in 70.00% of cases, the carer reports that it is the nurses who carry out this procedure, thus demonstrating that there are people with specialised professions for this procedure.

They also report that in 46.66 per cent of cases, the staff at the institutions already knew how to carry out this procedure, and in 10 per cent of cases the mother went to the institution and taught them how to administer tube diets.

In these cases, we see that the mother carer is being a multiplier of the teachings passed on to her.

5.3 Household demand

Currently we can see that in 80.00% of cases patients are using a button-type probe (at skin level) while in 20.00% they are using a foley-type probe.

This shows the dynamics of changing probes in the outpatient clinic, as first we use the probe placed during surgery (Pezzer), which remains in place for around 3 months for the gastrostomy to heal. Then we use the foley tube for up to 2 months, and finally we put in the button tube, which was measured according to the patient's gastrostomy.

During this time, the carer is trained to handle the patient's tube, as well as caring for the patient's other needs.

However, we found that 46.00% of the carers don't remember what the Pezzer probe is like or what it was like to take care of it, because it was only used after surgery and when a problem occurs with the button or Pezzer probe, the

Foley probe is used until a new button probe is purchased, with no further contact with the Pezzer probe.

In relation to the foley tube, 76.00% of the carers have negative reports, while 94.00% of the reports referring to the button tube are positive, and so it can be concluded from these statements that 92.00% prefer the button tube, which can also be seen in the statements by Matugama et al who say: "Silicone devices with a unidirectional valve (Willson-Cook®, Mik-Key®, PEG/FLOW®, BARD. Button®, Genie®, Tri-funnel®, Wizard®) are selected according to the consistency of the diet and the thickness of the abdominal wall in order to promote total adaptation: Button®, Genie®, Ponsky®, Tri-funnel®, Wizard®) are selected according to the consistency of the diet and the thickness of the abdominal wall, in order to promote total adaptation, preventing leaks and therefore dispensing with the use of skin protection plates, as complications are rare and the device can be changed every 6 or 8 months or when the valve has a problem. [85]

With regard to the training sessions held at HEB (Bauru State Hospital) for tube care, in 88.00% of the cases, the carers reported that they had taken part; with regard to training in handling diets, 92.00% reported that they had taken part and 80.00% of these carers said that the guidance was sufficient. However, as Heyman and et al point out: "carers of children with chronic illnesses require a great deal of time and effort to be trained and subsequently to provide the necessary care for their children. The carer must be knowledgeable about the child's illness and general condition and qualified to provide the necessary support, both technical and emotional, required by these children".[65]

One of the most worrying complications is the removal of the gastrostomy tube and how the carers behaved in the face of this; 84.00% of the carers said that the tube was removed at home, of these, 45.23% went to an emergency service to replace the tube, but 33.33% replaced the tube and then went to a health service. [86]

In 72% of cases, the carers reported that the tube's balloon had ruptured, making it easier for the tube to come out. In these cases, the outpatient clinic's advice is that if there is any complication that causes the tube to come out, it should be sanitised and repositioned immediately, avoiding closure of the gastrostomy, which occurs quickly in most patients, as we can see from Ruiz et al "in the event of accidental or intentional removal of the tube, the priority will be to avoid its closure and although access to the hospital or clinic or the necessary equipment is available, you can place the Foley tube with the inflated balloon in the lumen of the gastric region".[86]

When using the Foley tube, 58.00% of the carers reported that it had entered the stomach, as we can correlate with table 2 in the introduction, which shows tube migration and its implications[20] . In this case, the training given to the carer should be taken into account, as they were taught to keep the Foley tube fixed with adhesive tape and if it entered the stomach it should not be pulled out, as this could cause further injury, but they should go to the health service to have the balloon deflated and repositioned correctly.

Another complaint made by 44.00% of carers is related to leakage from the gastrostomy, even if the balloon is filled correctly, as we have already shown in table 4 of the introduction to this study[7] ; this problem can cause skin irritation and should be monitored with dressings to prevent further injury. [86]

As for skin lesions, 68.00% of the carers reported them around the gastrostomy area, as Landis et al point out: "ostomy can help cure the disease and even save lives, but sometimes complications occur and the most common complication is peristomal dermatitis". Of these cases, 47.05% cleaned well and used (non-specific) ointments and 20.59% used substances that could further damage the site, such as alcohol. The need for greater monitoring of this type of problem is therefore evident. [87]

As for the difficulty in administering diets, 84.00% of the cases reported no difficulties, while 50.00% of those who did experience some difficulty were when changing their diet and administering thick medication.

90.00% of the diets are industrialised and can be obtained from 70.00% of town halls, which facilitates the family routine and the carer's dynamic, avoiding time spent preparing homemade diets.

In 68.00% of the patients, the amount in millilitres of each diet was around 100 ml. to 200 ml. and with regard to the time taken to administer the diet, 26.00% of the carers reported that they used a time of approximately 15 min. to 30 min. and 28.00% of the carers used a time of 40 min. to 55 min.

In these cases, the statistics used (Pearson's correlation), in relation to the millilitres of diets for each administration at the times reported (p= 0.03 and R= -0.30), show that, as the quantity (volume) of diets increases, the administration time decreases, which causes diarrhoea and vomiting, as shown in table 4 of the introduction to this research, indicating that immediate action should be taken to reduce administration, in order to avoid these problems. [7]

According to the author Cappellano, "the feeding technique for the best nutrition of the neuropathic child should be slow and prolonged so as not to alter the pressure of the lower oesophageal sphincter tone, avoiding the possibility of reflux".[88]

Table 5 shows that the majority of patients gained weight within 6 months of surgery and Table 6, which shows height measurements within 6 months of surgery, shows that 10 patients grew and 6 patients remained the same height.

Therefore, with the aid of gastrostomy, better dietary provision contributes to the child's development and as Stenvenson et al report "nutrition is an important area for treatment of children with cerebral palsy and it is imperative to clarify the role of nutrition in maintaining health and well-being. Evidence documenting the effects of malnutrition on the poor growth and health of children with cerebral palsy is limited. Although much of the research has been done on adults and children without disabilities, it is applicable to this population. The adverse effects of malnutrition on physiology, motor function, neurological and psychological function are wide-ranging and can be particularly devastating in early development."[55]

In charts 7 and 8, we can see that most carers don't follow the guidelines correctly when it comes to using cleaning products on the probes and extensions, and when it comes to packaging the extensions, they also act in the same way, i.e. they use and store them as they see fit, which means that the product in the button-type probe, which is made of silicone, is quickly damaged and can't withstand the normal expected time of use, which is 9 months, so it has to be replaced early on several occasions in order to meet the patient's needs. This is clear from the carers' complaints, seen in chart 9, that they want more probes in less time.

However, this request is jeopardised by the caregivers' improper maintenance of the probes, since they are being cleaned and packaged in a way that goes against what is recommended by this clinic.

Within this approach, Motti and Kavalco state that "counselling is an element of family support from health professionals that raises the levels of perception of family members in relation to the child's problem [89,90].

And so, as Leite and Prado point out, "the importance of an orientation programme, because when well oriented, the caregiver can properly direct the care they give to the child and contribute to the rehabilitation process at home". [91]

CHAPTER 6

CONCLUSION

In view of the proposed objectives, the results obtained in this study led to the following conclusions:

- In characterising the sample, 60.00% of the 50 patients were female. The predominant age group (32.00%) was 6 to 10 years old, followed by 11 to 15 years old (24.00%), 2 to 5 years old (22.00%), 16 to 18 years old (6.00%) and over 18 years old (16.00%). The average age of the patients in the study was 11.43 years ± (standard deviation 6.52). 70.00% were white. The main medical diagnosis was cerebral palsy (100.00%), 92.00% of the patients had undergone surgical gastrostomy and due to dysphagia 72.00% did not use oral feeding. The main nutritional diagnosis was malnutrition (91.17%).

- In characterising the 50 carers, 98.00% were female and 2.00% male. The average age was 40.82 years ± (standard deviation 11.01), with a minimum of 25 years and a maximum of 70 years. The majority were white, 70.00%. Most of the carers were related to the mother (86.00%). The average family income in minimum wages is 2.32 ± minimum wages per family (standard deviation is 1.02), with a maximum value of 7.82 minimum wages. All of them live in houses with running water and electricity and the majority have a house with a slab 56.00%. The majority live on the outskirts 52.00% and 72.00% use public transport.

- As for the difficulties encountered, the majority (84.00%) reported that the tube came out of the ostomy, with reports of emesis (44.00%) after the tube was inserted, and the majority (68.00%) of skin lesions. The most common intercurrence (72.00%) was the rupture of the tube's balloon (Foley or button) and the entry of the Foley tube into the stomach in 58.00% of cases.

It is clear that although the service offers a fairly adequate care structure, with a multidisciplinary team to meet the different and complex demands of patients and their families, there is still a need to review health education strategies.

CHAPTER 7

BIBLIOGRAPHICAL REFERENCES

1. Santos JS,l Kemp R, Sankarankutty AK, Junior WS, Tirapelli LF, Júnior OCS .Gastrostomy and jejunostomy: aspects of technical evolution and expansion of indications. Medicina (Ribeirão Preto) 2011;44(1):39-50

2. Waitzberg DL. Oral, enteral and parenteral nutrition in clinical practice, 3rd EDITION. PART 6 PAGE 561 A734, 2002

3. Matsubara MGS, Villela DL, Hashimoto SY, Reis HCS. Wounds and Stomas in Oncology: an interdisciplinary approach.1ª ed. São Paulo: Ed. Lemar; 2012.

4. McGeer AJ, Detsky AS, Rourke KO. Parenteral nutrition in patients receiving cancer chemotherapy. American College of Physicians. Ann Intern Ned 1989; 110: 734-6.

5. Sena MJ, Utter GH, Cuschieri J, Maier RV, Tompkins RG, Harbrecht BG, More EE, O'Keefe GE. Early supplemental parenteral nutrition is associated with increased infectious complications in critically ill trauma patients. Jam Coll Surg 2008; 207(4): 459-67.

6. Griffiths R. Parenteral nutrition in adult inpatients with functioning gastrointestinal tracts: assessment of outcoes. Lancet 2006; 367 (9516): 1101-1111.

7. Ruiz ABF, Castillo SG, Lucendo AJ. Perctal endoscopic gastroscopy: an update on indications, technique and nursing care. Enferm Clin. 2011; 21(3): 173-178.

8. Minicucci MF et al. The use of percutaneous endoscopic gastrostomy. Ver Nut [on line] 2005;18(4): 553-559.

9. Gauderer MW, Ponsky JL, Izant RJ. Gastrostomy without laparotomy: a percutaneous endoscopic technique. J Paediatr Surg 198; 15(6): 872-5

10. Smeltzer SC, Bare BG.Treatise on medical-surgical nursing. 9th ed. Rio de Janeiro, RJ: Guanabara Koogan AS, 2002

11. Okano N, et al. Gastrostomy closure.Acta Cir Brás [on line] 2000; 15(2): 103-104

12. Townsend CM, Beauchamp RD, Evers BM, Mattox KL.Sabiston Treatise on Surgery.17ª ed. Texas: Saunders Elsevier; 2005)

13. Grant DG, Bradley PT, Pothier DD, Bailey D, Caldera S, Baldwin DL, Birchall MA.Complications following gastrostomy tube insertion in patients with head and neck cancer: a prospective multi-institution study, systematic review and meta-analysis.Clin Otolaryngol 2009; 34(2):103-112.

14. Stamm M. Gastrostomy withaout; a new method. Med News1894; 65:324-326.

15. Hashiba K. Endoscopic gastrostomy. Endoscopy 1987; 19(1):23- 4.

16. Chen HL, Shih SC, Bair MJ, Lin IT, Wu CH. Percutaneous Endoscopic Gastrotomy in the enteral feeding of the elderly. Inter J Geront. 2011; 5:135-138

17. Pelosof AG. Percutaneous endoscopic gastrostomy. In: Kowalski, Luiz Paulo et al. Manual de condutas diagnósticas e terapêuticas em oncologia. 2 ed. São Paulo: Âmbito Editores, 2002. p. 156-159

18. Souza JCK. Paediatric surgery - theory and practice. ia ed. São Paulo: Ed Roca Ltda.; 2007

19. Phillips TE, Cornejo CJ, Hoffer EK, McCormick WC. Gastrostomy and jejunostomy placement: The urban hospital perspective pertinent to nursing home care. J Am Med Dir Assoc. 2005;6: 390-395

20.   Brewster BD, Weil BR, Ladd AP. Prospective Determination of percutaneous endoscopic gastrostomy complication rates in children: Still a safe procedure. Surgery. 2012 oct, 152(4): 714-721

21.   Wiggenraad RGJ, Flierman L, Goossens A, Brand R, Verschuur HP, Croll GA, Moser LEC, Vriesendorp R. Prophylactic gastrostomy placement and early tube feeding may limit loss of weight during chemoradiotherapy for advanced head and neck cancer, a preliminary

study. Clin Otolaryngol 2007; 32(5):384-90

22.   Ruiz ABF, Castillo SG, Lucendo AJ. Percutaneous endoscopic gastrostomy: an update on indications, technique and nursing care.Enferm Clin. 2011; 21(3):173-178

23.   Perissé VLC. The nurse in caring for and teaching the family of the client with gastrostomy in the home setting. Niterói. Dissertation [master's degree in nursing] - Fluminense Federal University; 2007.

24.   Mello GFS, Mansur GR, Guimarães DP. Probes for ostomies. In [Various contributors]. Therapeutic Gastrointestinal Endoscopy.1ª ed. São Paulo: Tecmedd Editora; 2006.217-222

25.   Gauderer MWL, Picha GJ, Izant RJ. The gastrostomy button: a simple, skin-level, nonrefluxing device for long-term enteral feedings, J Pediat Surg 1984;19:803-5

26.   Diament A, Cypel S, reed UC. Child neurology.5th ed. São Paulo: Ed. Atheneu, 2010

27.   Rosemberg S. Neuropediatria.1st ed. São Paulo: Ed Sarvier, 1992

28.   Kinsbourne M, Batzdorf U, Gabriel RS, Weil ML. Treatise on neuropediatrics. 2nd ed.Los angeles: Ed Manole, 1984

29.   Yeargin-Allsop M, Braun KVN, Doernberg NS, Benedict RE, Kirby RS, Durkin MS. Prevalence of cerebral palsy in 8-year-old children in three areas of the United States in 2002: a multisite collaboration. Pediatrics 2008;121:547-554 [PubMed: 18310204].

30.   Christensen E, Melchior J. Cerebral palsy. A clinical and neuropathological study.Clinics in Developmental Medicine, n.25.London: W Heinemann, 1967.

31.   Stevenson R. Beyond growth: gastrostomy feeding in children with cerebral palsy. Developm medic and child neurol 2005, 47: 76-76

32.   Kuperminc MN, Stevenson RD. Growth and nutrition disorders in children with cerebral palsy. Dev Disabil Res Rev. 2008; 14(2): 137-146

33.   Rugiu MG.Role of videofluoroscopy in evaluation of neurologic dysphagia. Acta Otorhinolaryngol Ital. 2007; 27:306-316

34.   Dematteo C, Matovich D, Hjartarson A. Comparison of clinical and videofluoroscopic evaluation of children with feeding and swallowing difficulties. Develop Med and Child Neurol. 2005,47:149-157

35.   Silva SVS, Schmidt AFS, Mezzacappa MA, Marba ST, Siva JMB, Sbragia L. Babies with brain damage who cannot swallow. Arq Neuropsiquiatr. 2008; 66(3-b): 641-645

36.   Gaut, D.Development of a theoretically adequate description of caring. Western Journal of Nursing Resaerch, v.5, n.4, p.313-324, 1983

37.   Rossi, MSJ, Espaço, poder e saúde: a reforma Carlos Chagas [Free Teaching Thesis] Rio de Janeiro. University of Rio de Janeiro. Alfredo Pinto Nursing School, 1991. 471p

38.   Angelo M, Bousso, RS. Seeking to preserve the integrity of the family unit: the family living the experience of having a child in the ICU. Rev. Esc. Enf. USP, 2001 Jun, v.35, n.2, p. 172-9

39.   Menzies I. O funcionamento das organizações como sistemas sociais de defesa contra a ansiedade..São Paulo, Escola de Administração de Empresas da FGV.s.d. (mimeographed) 1979:1-50

40.   Leite NSL, Cunha SR. The family of the technology-dependent child: fundamental aspects for nursing practice in the hospital environment; Esc Anna Nery R Enferm 2007 Mar;11(1):92-7

41.   Romão CP, Almeida SB, Ponce de Leon CGRM. Gastrostomised patients: coping of caregivers at home. Rev Elet Enferm UNIEURO, Brasília,2008 v.1, n.2:18-34

42.   Souza LL,Gomes GC, Barros EJL. Caring for people with ostomies: the role of the family carer; Rev Enferm. UERJ, Rio de Janeiro, 2009 Oct/Dec; 17(4): 550-5.2).

43.   Pinto JP, Ribeiro CA, Pettengill MM, Balieiro MMFG. Family-centred care and its application in paediatric nursing. Rev Brás Enferm.

Brasília 2010 jan-feb; 63(1): 132-135

44.	Almeida, Maria Inez et al. Being the mother of a child with a chronic illness: carrying out complex care. Esc. Anna Nery [on line]. 2006, vol. 10, n. 1, pp.36-46. ISSN 1414-8145)

45.	Blum RW. Improving transition for adolescents with special health care needs from paediatric to adultcentered health care.[published correction appears pediatrics 2003;111:449]. Pediatrics 2002; 110(6 suppl): 1301-35

46.	Goldson E, Louch G, Washington K, Scheu H. Guidelines for the care of the child with special health care needs. Adv Paediatr. 2006, 53: 165-182

47.	Gomes ILV, Caetano R, Jorge MSB. Mothers' understanding of the care provided by the healthcare team in a children's hospital. Rev Bras Enferm. Brasília 2010 jan-feb; 63(1): 84-90

48.	Moore CP, Frizzell J, Richmond A, Copeland K. Nursing and equipment troubleshooting for special needs children in the emergency department.Elsevier Inc. 2012; 13(2): 133-141

49.	Mesman GR, Kuo DZ, Carroll JL, Ward WL.The impact of technology dependence on children and their families. J Ped H Care. 2012,may :1-9 [doi:10.1016/j.pedhc.2012.05.003

50.	Rabello CAFG, Rodrigues PHA. Family health and children's palliative care: listening to family members of technology-dependent children; ciência e saúde coletiva, 15(2):379-388, 2010.

51.	Waldow, VR. Moment of care: a moment of reflection on action: Rev. Bras. enferm, brasília 2009; jan-feb;62(1):140-5

52.	Bocchi SCM. The role of nurses as educators with family carers of people with strokes. Rev.bras. Enferm. 2004 Sept./Oct, Br,vol.57 no. 5

53.	Peduzzi M. Equipe multiprofissional de saúde: conceito e typologia. Rev. Saúde Pub. 2001;35(1):103-9

54.	Peduzzi M. Equipe multiprofissional de saúde: a interface entre trabalho e interação.[Tese].Campinas: Faculdade de Ciências Médicas, Universidade estadual de Campinas; 1998.

55.   Kuperminc MN, Stevenson RD. Growth and Nutrition Disorders in Children with Cerebral Palsy. Dev Disabil Res Rev. 2008; 14(2): 137146.

56.   Samson-Fang L, Fung E, Stallings VA, et al. Relationship of nutritional status to health and societal participation in children with cerebral palsy. J Pediatr 2002;141:637-643 [PubMed: 12410191]

57.   Stevenson RD, Conaway M, Chumlea WC, et al. Growth and health in children with moderate-to-severe cerebral palsy. Pediatrics 2006b;118:1010—1018. [PubMed: 16950992]

58.   Gomez, F. Et al. Mortality in second and third degree malnutriton.Journal of Tropical Paediatrics. V.2, p.77-83, 1956.

59.   Waterlow, C. Et al.The presentation and use of height and weight data for comparing the nutritional status of groups of chidren under the age of 10 years. Bulletin of the World Health Organisation. V.55, n.44, p. 489-498, 1977.

60.   Brazilian Paediatric Society. Nutritional assessment of children and adolescents - Guidance Manual / Brazilian Paediatric Society. Department of Nutrology. - São Paulo: Brazilian Society of Paediatrics. Department of Nutrology, 2009,

61.   krick, J. et al. Pattern of growth in children with cerebral palsy. Journal of the American Dietetic Associaton. V.96, n°7,p.680-685.July,1996.

62.   National Health Council. Resolution 196, of October 1996. Guidelines and Regulatory Norms for Research Involving Human Beings. Brasília, Ministry of Health; 1996)

63.   Bauru State Hospital. AIPEG Standards and Routines Manual. São Paulo: HEB; 2011.

64.   Wu YW, Colford JM. Chorioamnionitis as a risk factor for cerebral palsy. JAMA 2000;284:1414-7

65. Heyman MB, Harmatz P, Acree M, Wilson L, Moskowitz JT, Ferrando S, Folkman S. Economic and psychologic costs for maternal caregivers of gastrostomy-dependent children. The J Ped.2004 Oct; 145: 511-516

66. Nicholl HM, Begley CM. Explaining caregiving by mothers of children with complex needs in Ireland: A Phenomenological study. J Ped Nurs. 2012; 27: 642-651

67. Kirk S, Glendinning C. Supporting 'expert' parents-professional suort and families caring for a child with complex health care needs in the community. Inter J N S. 2002; 39: 625-635

68. Machado ALG, Jorge MSB, Freitas CHA. The experience of the family carer of a stroke victim: an interactionist approach. Rev Bras Enferm. Brasília 2009 Mar-Apr; 62(2): 246-25

69. Cabral, IE.Being a mother and the re-discovery of knowledge in the natural stimulation of her children[Dissertation].Rio de Janeiro: Anna Nery Nursing School.UFRJ.1994

70. Susin FP, Bortolini V, Sukiennik R, Mancopes R, Barbosa BLDR. Profile of patients with cerebral palsy using gastrostomy and effect on carers. Rev. CEFAC. 2012 Sep-Oct; 14(5):933-942

71. Costa VV, Saraiva RA, Torres RVD, TSA, Oliveira SB. Action of anticonvulsants alone and associated with midazolam as pre-anaesthetic medication on Bispectral Indices (BIS) in patients with cerebral palsy. Rev Brás Anestesiol 2010; 60(3): 259-267.

72. IBGE, National Household Sample Survey 2003

73. Complete mortality tables. Rio de Janeiro: IBGE, 2008. Available at: <http://www.ibge.gov.br/servidor_arquivos_est>. Accessed on: June 2009.

74. Margre ALM, Reis MGL, Morais RLS. Characterisation of adults with cerebral palsy. Rev Brás Fisiot, São Carlos 2010, v.14, n.5, p. 417-25

75. Milbrath VM, Amestoy SC, SoaresDC, Siqueira HCH.

Comprehensiveness and accessibility in the care of children with cerebral palsy. Acta Paul Enferm 2009; 22(6): 755-760

76. Fung EB, Samson-Fang l, Stallings VA, et al. Feeding dysfunction is associeated with poor growth and health status in children with CP.J Am Diet Assoc 2002; 102:361-373

77. Glat R, Duque MA.Convivendo com filhos especiais: o olhar paterno.5ª edition.Rio de Janeiro: Viveiros de Castro;2003.

78. Strauss D, Brooks J, Shavelle R. Life expectancy in cerebral palsy: an update. Dev Med Child Neurol. 2008;50(7):487-93

79. Guimarães AQ, Wandreley BC. Project to evaluate Minas Gerais in the first years of the 21st century - report on the economic and social areas - second half of 2006. Belo Horizonte: João Pinheiro Foundation; 2006.

80. Sleigh G, Brocklehurst P. Gastrostomy feeding in cerebral palsy: a systematic review.Arch Dis Child 2004;89:534-539

81. Sullivan PB, Juszczak E, Bachlet AM, et al.Gastrostomy tube feeding in children with cerebral palsy: a prospective, longitudinal study. Dev Méd Child Neurol 2005;47:77-85

82. O'Neill JK, O'Neill PJ, Goth-Owens T, Horn B, Cobb LM. Caregiver evaluation of anti-gastroesophageal reflux procedures in neurologically impaired children: what is the real-life outcome? J Pediatr Surg 1996; 31:375-380.

83. Fonkalsrud EW, Ashcraft KW, Coran AG, et al. Surgical treatment of gastroesophageal reflux in children: A combined hospital study of 7467 patients. Paediatrics 1998; 101:419-422.

84. Enumo, SRF. Assisted assessment for children with special educational needs: an auxiliary resource for school inclusion.Rev Bras Educ Esp;11(3):335-354, Sep.-Dec. 2005.

85. Matugama S, Ishioka S.Endoscopic gastrostomy and jejunostomy. In Sakai P, Ishioka S, Maluf Filho F. Tratado de endoscopia digestiva e terapêutica - estomago e duodeno. São Paulo: Atheneu; 2001.p297-306.

86.   Ruiz ABF, Castillo SG, Lucendo AJ. Percutaneous endoscopic gastrostomy: an update on indications, technique and nursing care.Enferm Clin. 2011; 21(3):173-178

87.   Landis MN, Keeling JH, Yiannias JA, Richardson DM, Lenehan DLN, Davis MDP.Results of patch testing in 10 patients with peristomal dermatitis. J Am Acad Dermatol 2012 Sep; 67(3):92-104

88.   Cappellano G. Gastrostomy and gastroesophageal reflux in neuropathic children. Einstein.2003;1:117-123

89.   Motti, T. M. F. (2005). A non-presential counselling programme for parents of hearing-impaired children. PhD thesis, Federal University of São Carlos, São Paulo, Brazil.

90.   Kavalco, T. F. (2003). The effectiveness of functional seated positioning guidelines applied at home to family members of a child with cerebral palsy: A case study. Unpublished monograph, State University of Western Paraná, Paraná, Brazil.

91.   Leite, J. M. R., & Prado, G. F. (2004). Cerebral palsy: Physiotherapeutic and clinical aspects. Revista Neurociências, 12, 41-45.

8 APPENDIX

1.1 Appendix 1: Informed consent form

(Mandatory terminology in compliance with resolution 196/96 - CNS-MS)

Name:_______________________________________Age:_______ ID: _________

I invite you to take part in the project: "Profile of children treated at a gastrostomy outpatient clinic and the demands and difficulties in home care", developed by me, Ana Cristina Ferreira Martins, a nurse at Bauru State Hospital and a regular student on the professional master's degree course at Unesp Botucatu, which aims to analyse the difficulties in home care, according to the profile of patients with gastrostomies, by means of a questionnaire with questions about the care and demands inherent in this care.

The interview will be held at the outpatient clinic and will take an average of 40 minutes, at the end of which guidance will be given according to the carer's doubts and complaints.

I would like to make it clear that the study will not cause any embarrassment or risk, and that you are free to refuse to take part or to leave the study at any time without any personal harm, and that your name will be kept strictly confidential when the results of the research are published.

This form will be signed in two copies, one of which will remain in your possession and the other will be the responsibility of the researcher.

I am at your disposal at any time for clarification if necessary.

If you have any further questions, please contact the Research Ethics Committee on (14) 3811-6143.

I am hereby _________________________________ duly informed, I hereby give my free and informed consent, agreeing to take part in the proposed research. I have also received a copy of this consent form.

Bauru, ___ // __

ResearcherPatient

Ana Cristina Ferreira Martins / regular Master's student-UNESP/Botucatu
Phone: (14) 3284 59 82 / e-mail: acf martins@yahoo.com.br

1.2 Appendix 2: Patient profile questionnaire

1. Patient registration
2. Age
3. Sex
4. Colour
5. City of Origin
6. Medical Diagnosis:
7. Date of joining AIPEG
8. Date of surgery
9. Days of hospitalisation during surgery

10. Type of Surgery (gastrostomy and without/with valve)

11. Estimated weight and height at the first AIPEG consultation.

12. Estimated weight and height on return to the outpatient clinic.

13. Estimated weight and height 4 months after surgery.

14. Nutritional assessment:

a) Interpretation:

1ª consultation ( ) Post-surgery return:( ) 4 months post-surgery:( )

b) Nutritional Diagnosis:

1consultation ( ) Return post-surgery( ) 6 months post-surgery( )

1.3 Appendix 3: Home care demand survey I - IDENTIFICATION

15) Patient's name:

16) Hospital ID:

17) age:

18) sex:

19) colour:

20) Father's name :

21) Mum's name:

22) Name of main carer:

23) colour of the carer:

24) age of the main carer:

25) Main carer's profession:

26) Degree of kinship with the patient:

27) Level of education of the carer:

( )Illiterate

( )1st degree complete

( )2nd degree complete

( ) Complete 3rd degree

( )other

II - Family:

28) No. of family members and their ages:

( ) Children --- 0 to 1 year ( )quantities

------------------------------------- 1 to 3 years( ) quantities   3

to 5 years( ) quantities --------- 5 to 7 years( ) quantities   7

to 12 years( ) quantities ------- 12 to 18 years( ) quantities

( ) Adults18 --------------------------------- to 25 years old( ) quantities

-------------------------------------25 to 45 years old( ) quantities

------------------------------- 45 to 60 years old( ) quantities

( ) Elderly ----------------------------------- 60 to 70 years old( ) quantities

------------------------------- 70 more( ) quantities

29)Family income: ____ .

III - HOUSING

30)Housing conditions:

( )own residence

( )rental home

( )other

31)Number of rooms in the house:

32)Piped water: ( )Yes ( )No

33)Cemented floor: ( )Yes ( )No

34)Electric light: ( )Yes ( )No

35)Construction: ( )Brick house ( )Wooden house

36)Roof: ( )asbestos ( )ceramic ( )slab

37)City you live in:_________________________________

38)Neighbourhood: ( ) Centre ( ) Periphery

IV - TRANSPORT

39) Transport:

( ) Public

( ) Private

( ) Other

V - INSTITUTIONALISATION

40)Institutionalised child: ( ) yes ( ) no

41)Name of institution:_______________

42)City:_______________________________

43)Do you have trained nurses: ( ) Yes ( ) No

44)Accompanied by a nutritionist: ( ) Yes ( ) No

45)Accompanied by a doctor: ( ) Yes ( ) No

46)Reason for institutionalisation: ____

VI - SOUND

47)Since your son had surgery, which probe has he used?

Pezzer ( ) comment: ____

Foley ( ) comment: ____

Button ( ) comment: ____

48)Which probe does the child currently use? _____________________

49)Which do you prefer?

Comment: ____

VII - AFTER SURGERY

50)Were you trained to handle the probe after surgery?

    yes( ) no ( )

51)After surgery, were you trained to handle the diet preparations?

    yes( ) no ( )

52)Until you returned to the gastrostomy clinic, were the guidelines you were given enough for you to take care of yourself?

    Yes ( ) No ( )

53)Comment: ____

VIII- COMPLICATIONS AT HOME:

54)What were the complications and what did you do about each one?

55) ( ) Probe exit, and I did _________________________________

56) ( )Diarrhoea, and I did_________________________________

57) ( )Aspiration, and I did _________________________________

58) ( )Vomiting, and I did_____________________

59) ( )Reflux, and I did ___________________________

60) ( )Obstruction, and I did ___________________________

61) ( )Break extensions, and I did___________________________

62) ( )Difficulties in preparing diets, and I did ___________________

63) ( )Bruise around the skin, and I did___________________________

IX - SUPPLY ROUTES

64)Is your child exclusively on a tube diet?

        Yes ( )   no ( )

65)Is your child cleared for oral feeding?

        Yes ( )   no ( )

66)What should be done with the tube after the diet?

67)What should be done with the extensions after the diet?

68)Have you ever had difficulty passing the diet? ( ) yes ( ) no

69)At what point? ____

70)How was it? ____

71)What kind of diet do you use? ___________________________________

72)Where do you buy the diet?___________________________________

73)How many ml do you provide in each diet? ___________________

74)What position does the child need to be in to start the diet?

75)How long should the diet be administered?

X - OTHER

76)How do you take your medication?

XI - COMPLICATIONS WITH PROBES

77)Has the probe balloon ever burst?

78)When this happened, what did you do the 1ª time?

79)And today, if the balloon pops, do you know what to do?

80)When your child used the Foley tube, did it "go into" the stomach?

81)Did you realise when the probe went into your stomach?

82)What do you do to stop the tube going into your stomach?

XII - SKIN COMPLICATIONS

83)Have you ever damaged the skin around the probe?

( ) Yes ( ) No

84)If so, how many times has this happened?

85)What did you do? ________________________________

XII - GASTROSTOMY LEAKS

86)Does it leak? ( )Yes ( ) No

87)What do you do?

88)When does the diet usually leak through the gastrostomy?

XIII - CLEANING THE PROBE

89)When and how do you clean the probe?

90)What do you use to clean?

91)How do you store the button probe extensions?

92) Do you remove the button probe for cleaning?( )Yes ( )No

93)Does the child belong to an institution?

94)Is she fed during this period?

95)Who feeds her?

96)Who taught her how to feed?

97-Did you have any difficulties that weren't mentioned or asked about that you'd like to report?

8.4 Appendix 4: Tables

Chart 5: Patients' weight change in relation to 1ª outpatient appointment and up to 6 months after surgery.

Database registration	Age when you had surgery	Weight 1ª consultation	Weight after 6 months	Amendment
4	10 months	7,4	8	Increased
5	2	7,9	12,25	Increased
20	1	8,05	7,5	Decreased
23	1	7,33	7,79	Increased
24	2	12,1	11,65	Decreased

31	6 months	3,84	6,58	Increased
36	1	12,2	18,45	Increased
39	1	8,13	9,4	Increased
43	1	7,56	9,48	Increased
45	1	7,47	9,6	Increased
50	1	No annotation	No annotation	**********
7	3	11,1	12,8	Increased
11	5	22,25	24	Increased
19	5	No annotation	15	**********
26	3	13,27	15,55	Increased
1	10	15,95	17,45	Increased
8	10	20,5	25	Increased
14	9	17,2	20,5	Increased
28	6	No annotation	No annotation	**********
30	7	16k	22,6	Increased
34	7	17	21	Increased
38	6	11,8	15,6	Increased
41	8	18	19,4	Increased
42	7	12,4	14,75	Increased
46	10	15,7	18,5	Increased
47	6	11,75	14,33	Increased
12	14	15,5	20	Increased
21	12	23,8	24,35	Increased
33	11	No annotation	No annotation	**********
35	15	15,9	18,9	Increased
37	11	11,05	12,6	Increased
49	15	21	21	Maintained
48	16	25,1	25,12	Maintained
2	21	No annotation	No annotation	**********
3	20	30	35,7	Increased

Chart 6: Patients' change in height in relation to their first visit to the outpatient clinic up to 6 months after surgery

Database registration	Age when you had surgery	Height 1º consultati	Height after 6 months	Amendmen

		on		t
4	10 months	82,1	90	Increased
5	2	No annotation	98	**********
20	1	81	81	Maintained
23	1	No annotation	76	**********
24	2	No annotation	102	**********
31	6 months	No annotation	68,2	**********
36	1	87,5	102	Increased
39	1	No annotation	No annotation	**********
43	1	No annotation	78	**********
45	1	No annotation	75	**********
50	1	No annotation	No annotation	**********
7	3	No annotation	89	**********
11	5	No annotation	121	**********
19	5	No annotation	No annotation	**********
26	3	No annotation	No annotation	**********
1	10	115	115	Maintained
8	10	140	140	Maintained
14	9	124	129	Increased
28	6	No annotation	No annotation	**********
30	7	115	121	Increased
34	7	109	114	Increased
38	6	100	107	Increased
41	8	106	118	Increased
42	7	106	112	Increased
46	10	124	124	**********
47	6	No annotation	105	**********
12	14	117	117	**********

21	12	130	130	***********
33	11	No annotation	No annotation	**********
35	15	140	142	Increased
37	11	110	110	Maintained
49	15	120	120	Maintained
48	16	141	141	Maintained
2	21	No annotation	No annotation	**********
3	20	149	156	Increased

Chart 7: Occurrence of variables in relation to the packaging of extension cords after use.

Recommends	Plastic container closed and placed in the cupboard (28)	Closed plastic container placed on top of the ice-cream maker. (1)	Closed plastic container on the kitchen table. (1)		Closed plastic container on top of the sink. (3)	
Not recommended	Product box (1)	Plastic container placed in the fridge (5)	Plastic container with water on top of the sink. (1)	Plastic container with closed lid in the child's bag. (1)	Container with water and bleach locked in the cupboard. (1)	Canister with dust guard on the table. (1)
No answer	No answer (2)					
Part of the process is missing	Plastic container (2)	Plastic container on top of the sink. (2)	Plastic container on top of chest of drawers (1)	Canister with cloth (1)	Canister with cloth in the cupboard. (1)	
Use another probe	Use Foley (5)					

Table 8: Occurrence of the variables in relation to the cleaning products used in the button probe and their extensions .

<table>
<tr>
<td>Recomen given</td>
<td colspan="2">Neutral detergent (11)</td>
<td>Neutral detergent and water (1)</td>
<td>Water and soap. (1)</td>
<td>Neutral detergent and cold water. (6)</td>
<td>Neutral detergent and coloured water.</td>
<td>Running water and detergent</td>
</tr>
<tr>
<td></td>
<td colspan="2"></td>
<td></td>
<td></td>
<td></td>
<td>(1)</td>
<td>neutral (1)</td>
</tr>
<tr>
<td rowspan="2">Not recommended</td>
<td>Hot water(1)</td>
<td>Running water and distilled water (1)</td>
<td>Sabonete (1)</td>
<td>Sanitary water</td>
<td>Neutral detergent and warm water</td>
<td>Warm, cold water with neutral soap</td>
<td>Boric water</td>
</tr>
<tr>
<td colspan="2">Use a knitting needle.</td>
<td>Distilled water and saline solution.</td>
<td>Saline solution.(3)</td>
<td>Running water and saline solution</td>
<td>Detergent serum and cold water.</td>
<td>Detergente, cold and hot water.</td>
</tr>
<tr>
<td>No answer u</td>
<td colspan="7">No answer (1)</td>
</tr>
<tr>
<td>Part of the process is missing</td>
<td colspan="2">Running water (5)</td>
<td>Filtered water (2)</td>
<td colspan="2">Cold water (1)</td>
<td colspan="2">With cold filtered water (1)</td>
</tr>
<tr>
<td>Don't know</td>
<td colspan="7">Doesn't know (1)</td>
</tr>
<tr>
<td>Use another probe</td>
<td colspan="4">Use Foley (5)</td>
<td colspan="3">(1)</td>
</tr>
</table>

TABLE 9: Openness to the carer about any complaints that were not asked about and that they would like to raise.

<table>
<tr>
<th>DOESN'T WANT TO COMMENT</th>
<th>SUPPLY OF MATERIALS: PROBE</th>
<th>AIPEG'S POSITIVE ASPECT</th>
<th>NEGATIVE ASPECTS OF AIPEG</th>
<th>THE CARER'S FEELINGS</th>
<th>DIFFICULTY GETTING AROUND</th>
<th>OTHER</th>
</tr>
<tr>
<td>I don't want to.
I don't want to.</td>
<td>Have a more resistant product and change it more times a year.</td>
<td rowspan="2">It's all good, but they could supply more rigs in the year.</td>
<td rowspan="2">AIPEG service takes too long from 7am to 12pm</td>
<td rowspan="2">At first I didn't sleep worrying about her pain</td>
<td rowspan="3">My municipality could change the probe so that I don't have to travel every month and wait for the ambulance all day.</td>
<td rowspan="2">I didn't find what I went through difficult and I'm hopeful that she'll remove the probe.</td>
</tr>
<tr>
<td>NO COMMENT</td>
<td>Extensions get dirty, very difficult to clean, need more kit in the year.</td>
</tr>
<tr>
<td></td>
<td>See suitable product for cleaning extensions, supply more probes and extensions.
The probes and extensions should be changed every 6 months,</td>
<td>I've always been well</td>
<td>I wish the service on the day of the group</td>
<td>I had a lot of fear (3) and difficulty sanitising.</td>
<td>I have difficulty brushing my teeth and back pain because I</td>
</tr>
</table>

because when they're old, they leak secretion and hurt the skin so you don't have to redo the gastrostomy.	looked after.	was quicker				have to carry it.
Change the probe and extension more often in a year.	Everything is fine, she's been attended to promptly every time she's needed it, and also with her needs with the probe.	Time-consuming group service	I wish I had family support, neighbours and people could call me and ask about him.	I'd like the driver to pick up the probe and bring it to my house for me to change.	I wanted to put my daughter in stem cell research.
The probe is very good, but the extension is very dirty and it's difficult to use the thicker extension.				Difficult to bring the child to appointments.	I'm afraid to handle it.
It's all good, but they could supply more rigs in the year.			I didn't want a gastrostomy, but I realised it was important.	I wanted to come to the hospital less because it's difficult and far away.	When there were no benefits, we were in need.
The probe gets very dirty, the extensions smell bad, I suggest changing the kit more often in the year and the diets should be more diluted and a container should be provided to store the extensions.	Everything's fine.				
They should change the probe and extensions every 6 months to improve hygiene and prevent the extensions from breaking.	Nothing is missing, I've always been well looked after.		I was terrified during a bath in hospital that I almost pulled the tube out because it got tangled.		Difficult to feed the child at first due to embarrassment
The probe needs to be changed more times a year because the extensions break.					
Change them more often in the year because they break easily(3)					
The time it takes to change the tube is too long, the extensions get dirty, break, clog when the tube gets old and the child ends up losing weight.					
I want more extensions in the kit because they damage and break					
Provide more extensions during the year.					

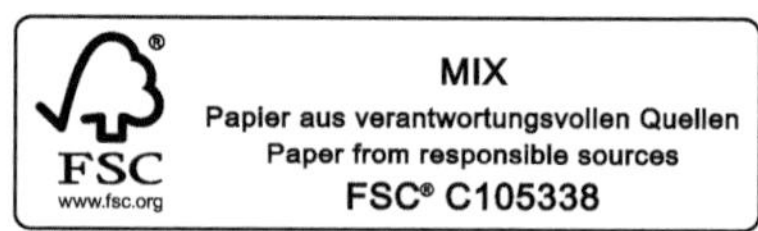

Printed by Books on Demand GmbH, Norderstedt / Germany